unhooked

Laura Dawn offers a refreshing new look at an ages old problem. She offers down to earth, sane solutions with no gimmicks. Working with nature as her guide, Laura Dawn combines science and common sense into a comprehensive and very effective program.

—Dr. Douglas Graham

Laura Dawn offers a holistic lifestyle-oriented approach to health and wellbeing that moves away from the old paradigm of "diet as deprivation" and helps support people to step into a sustainable and healthy lifestyle. This book will help you heal a disordered relationship with food to discover balance, health and happiness.

—Marcia Weider, CEO Dream University

You are about to begin a journey into understanding the very essence of what it means to be free from the known and unknown elements that have bound you to food, and enter into a lifetime adventure in exploring a loving relationship with yourself and all the ways in which you nurture every part of your being. Laura gently weaves the science of food, environment and all elements of Body, Mind and Spirit into a masterful flow of information that will uplift and guide you into a whole new realm of nutrition that goes far beyond just the food you eat."

—Lars Gustafsson, Founder and CEO: BodyMind Institute

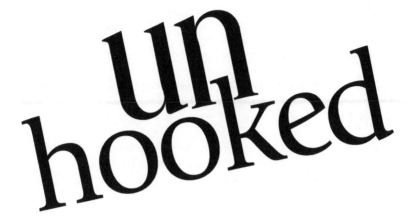

un hooked

a holistic approach to ending
YOUR *struggle with food*

laura dawn

NEW YORK

unhooked

a holistic approach to ending **YOUR** *struggle with food*

© 2015 Laura Dawn.

Published in New York, New York, by Morgan James Publishing. Morgan James and The Entrepreneurial Publisher are trademarks of Morgan James, LLC. www.MorganJamesPublishing.com

The Morgan James Speakers Group can bring authors to your live event. For more information or to book an event visit The Morgan James Speakers Group at www.TheMorganJamesSpeakersGroup.com.

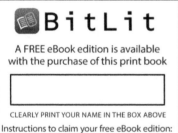

A FREE eBook edition is available with the purchase of this print book

CLEARLY PRINT YOUR NAME IN THE BOX ABOVE

Instructions to claim your free eBook edition:
1. Download the BitLit app for Android or iOS
2. Write your name in UPPER CASE in the box
3. Use the BitLit app to submit a photo
4. Download your eBook to any device

ISBN 978-1-63047-205-4 paperback
ISBN 978-1-63047-206-1 eBook
ISBN 978-1-63047-207-8 hardcover
Library of Congress Control Number: 2014935529

Cover Design by:
Rachel Lopez
www.r2cdesign.com

Interior Design by:
Bonnie Bushman
bonnie@caboodlegraphics.com

In an effort to support local communities, raise awareness and funds, Morgan James Publishing donates a percentage of all book sales for the life of each book to Habitat for Humanity Peninsula and Greater Williamsburg.

Get involved today, visit
www.MorganJamesBuilds.com

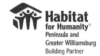

Habitat
for Humanity®
Peninsula and
Greater Williamsburg
Building Partner

Table of Contents

Acknowledgments   vii

Introduction: How We Get Hooked on the Food Struggle   ix

Part One: The Environmental Hook   1

Chapter 1   How Our Environment Hooks Us   3

Chapter 2   Unhooked: The Healing Process of Reconnection   22

Part Two: The Physiological Hook   39

Chapter 3   How Our Physiology Hooks Us   41

Chapter 4   Unhooked: Transitioning to a Whole Foods Lifestyle   58

Part Three: The Behavioral Hook   91

Chapter 5   How Our Behavioral Patterns Hook Us   93

Chapter 6   Unhooked: Committing to Change   104

Part Four: The Mental Hook   123

Chapter 7   How Our Mental State Hooks Us   125

Chapter 8   Unhooked: Learning to Eat Mindfully   135

Part Five: The Emotional Hook   155

Chapter 9   How Our Emotions Hook Us   157
Chapter 10   Unhooked: Working with Emotions and Boosting   168
                 the Feel-Good Chemicals in Your Brain Naturally

Part Six: The Spiritual Hook   181

Chapter 11   How Our Spiritual Isolation Hooks Us   183
Chapter 12   Unhooked: Deepening Your Spiritual Connection   191

Appendix A   Yale Food Addiction Scale   201
Appendix B   Understanding Fruit Sugars: Glycemic Index Versus 204
                 Glycemic Load
Appendix C   Basic Sitting Practice: Mindfulness-Awareness Meditation 206

                 About the Author   209
                 Endnotes   210

Acknowledgments

When I was in third grade, my math teacher told me I would never be good at math. Ironically, I went on to graduate with a business degree and a major in finance at the John Molson School of Business. Years later, after leaving the world of finance, as I was questing for my soul's desire, I sought advice from an intuitive healer. She told me in that conversation that I should never be a writer. Her voice likes to chime in at the back of my mind all too often, especially at the worst of moments. The truth is, I'm not a naturally talented writer, but what I do have are two very important things: a strong desire to help others free themselves from the food struggle, as I genuinely know what it's like to struggle so deeply, as well the support of incredibly loving people who have helped me every step of the way.

The one person who has always been there for me, through thick and thin, and who has gone to great lengths to help me see this project to completion, is my mother. I could not have asked to be born to anyone more loving and supportive than you. An entrepreneur, editor, and talented author—I humbly follow in your footsteps. I am also grateful to my father for raising me to believe in myself. You taught me that anything I can think up, I can achieve. It was this voice that would always counter the one saying I couldn't do it.

Thank you to my dear husband Noah—you have exemplified what it means to be in a loving, supportive marriage. Even before this book started to take shape, you believed in me. Thank you for working so hard to allow the space for me to write this book.

I would also like to give a special thank you to my ex-partner Keefer and his mother Manon. It was in your garden that I healed my relationship with food and changed my life forever. It was because of meeting you, Keefer, that I undertook this path.

Thank you to the Dream Queen herself: Marcia Wieder. You definitely helped make *this* dream come true, making this book a physical reality. You believed in me and supported me, and I will always be grateful for a dear friend like you. Amanda Rooker, my editor, also deserves a special thank you as you went above and beyond the call of duty and did a fantastic job helping me with this book.

Throughout the years I also had the support of my most cherished spiritual teachers in my life. Pema Chödrön, although I've never met you, I always carry you with me in my heart. You and your teachings have helped me get through the darkest moments of my life. I hope to some day thank you in person. Also, thank you to Wayne Dyer—yours were the first books on creating a new reality and understanding the power of intention that I read, many years ago now, and I refer back to them often. Thank you also to Dr. Douglas Graham. The "alternative" information and insights you've shared with me have forever changed and influenced my path. You've taught me how to be a more critical thinker and to not accept the status quo at face value. You truly are a revolutionary leader in the health and wellness movement.

I would also like to thank the many researchers and authors whom I quote, ranging from the science to the spiritual, all of whom helped lay the groundwork for me to continue to understand my own relationship with food.

Introduction

How We Get Hooked on the Food Struggle

It was day two of a weeklong retreat I was leading in Hawaii. The floor was now open for the workshop participants to share. I could feel the emotionally charged energy in the room as I waited patiently to see who would be the first to share. Silence.

A female participant sat quietly on the couch with a cushion over her lap, protection from feeling exposed. She hesitated to make eye contact and watched her hands twirl the frays on the corner of the cushion. "I think about food all the time," she finally offered in a low voice. "Thoughts about food and my weight consume me every day. I've tried so many different ways to be free of this struggle, but I can't seem to get over it. I've been using food to cope for as long as I can remember. I think about what I *want* to eat, what I *should* be eating, what I *shouldn't* be eating, *why* I shouldn't have eaten it. It makes me feel uncomfortable in my own skin, and I just want to hide." She paused. "I feel like there could be so much more to my life, like I'm holding myself down by continuously overeating. It makes me feel horrible, but

I don't know how to stop." The other participants sitting in the circle nodded their heads in silent agreement. They too knew what it was like to suffer in these silent ways. And so did I.

The food struggle that many of us engage in on a daily basis is invariably compounded by two debilitating factors: guilt and shame. Many people believe overeating implies moral weakness and failure, a complete lack of willpower and motivation, and the inability to "get a grip" on their eating habits. As a result, most people suffer in silence.

Two-thirds of the American population is either overweight or obese. Obviously many people struggle with overeating and all the consequences that go along with it. Although we've become accustomed to seeing oversized people everywhere, this is not normal, and this certainly wasn't the case as recently as thirty years ago. This is a collective dysfunctional situation, and it's no accident that it's happening. Even so-called "thin" people struggle with food addiction—chronically thinking about food, how much they weigh, and what diet they should try next, perhaps engaging in binge/purge cycles as I did for so many years.

My Journey Back Home to Myself

Although by outward appearances and society's standards I looked relatively healthy, few people knew the depths of my despair in my war against food and my body. My weight fluctuated with the predictable cycles of fierce, restrictive determination followed by a complete loss of control. I lost the weight and gained it back again . . . and again . . . and again. And my self-esteem fluctuated closely behind.

I desperately wanted—*needed*—to change, but I had tried countless times to "change"—only to follow mainstream advice that would inevitably lead me back to where I started—overeating, overweight, insecure, and depressed.

And I finally, inevitably, I hit rock bottom.

Looking back, it was a blessing in disguise. On my knees on the bathroom floor, gasping for air as I sobbed uncontrollably, I begged the Universe to help me—I knew with every cell in my body that there was more to my life than this.

And then, for a brief moment, I stopped crying, and somehow a window opened, providing a clear insight into the life I was living. I had been embarking on a highly "successful" path working in the finance industry and in that single moment I decided that this was no longer my life. It was like looking at myself through someone else's eyes and I could no longer identify with the person that I was. I knew this was the beginning of the most drastic change of my life: where I was living, who I was spending time with, what I was spending my time doing, and especially, the patterns around eating and food that I had perpetuated for so long. And in that precise revealing moment I decided to do the only logical thing I could think of—I left the only place I'd ever known to be home.

Once this comprehension had completely sunk in, there was no denying it's dynamic force. It was less of a decision than an internal awareness that this was what I *had* to do. Despite the fear of leaving, I knew without a shadow of a doubt that I had to embark on this path. As it turned out, it was the best decision I ever made. Trusting my intuition, no matter how uncomfortable it initially felt, has provided me with the most rewarding experiences in this life. I made the arrangements, gave up my apartment, and gave notice to work, friends, and family. I literally gave away or sold everything I owned, packed a backpack, and left. And I never went back.

I took a leap of faith into what seemed like the dark unknown, and the Universe responded in kind, as I believe it always does when that leap originates from a place of good intention. It has been an epic journey, one that has led me all over the world and ultimately back home to myself. I searched for answers to help me understand why I had spent most of my life struggling with food, my weight, and my*self,* and why I willingly chose to perpetuate patterns and behaviors that I knew made me unhealthy and unhappy.

Healed in a Garden

As I committed to healing my disordered relationship with food, my prayers were heard. I realized that I didn't want to wait until I was sixty years old and retired to spend more time in nature and learn how to grow a garden; I didn't want to wait to start living the life that I wanted to live now. So I started repeating an internal mantra: "I'm growing my own tomatoes . . . I'm ready to grow my own tomatoes." After I left home, I hitchhiked across British Columbia at the tender age of twenty-one, and I met a handsome smiling young man who was nice enough to give me a ride and spend the day with me before dropping me off at a quiet camping spot. I wouldn't see him again until one surprising day, six months later in a small town on the other side of the world, on a small island in Thailand. We fell in love and spent the next six years together.

Ironically, I moved home with him to a beautiful, 150-acre piece of land right near the same town where we had first met. I was taught by his whole family how to "live off the land" and grow my own food for the first time in my life. I will never forget the full-circle moment of deep insight into the power of our own will to heal, when I was walking up from the greenhouse that first summer with a basket filled with fifteen varieties of tomatoes. They were all so beautiful and unique and colorful, and tasted unlike any other store-bought tomato I had ever tried. It was the first moment that I realized I was living my mantra, growing my own tomatoes and living connected to my food source for the first time in my life. To some, the story might sound truly unbelievable, yet I now know that absolutely anything is possible when we have a clear, heartfelt intention. The state of my health—on all levels—was forever changed and the struggle was finally over.

It was in this garden that I tuned in to my own inherent wisdom and forever changed and healed my relationship with food, and what I had discovered was that I was actually connecting to something deeply sacred. My perception of food radically shifted as I realized the miracle that food truly is; something to love, not something to struggle with. I listened, watched, and trusted. My intuition strengthened, and I developed a strong sense of respect for nature. I realized that I too was (and always will be) a part of nature, intricately connected to the greater whole.

It was through this reconnection that it all started to make sense: the foods that I was hooked on, that kept me caught in the struggle, weren't *real, whole* foods from nature; they were processed food products made by food companies in a production plant. The longer I ate real, fresh, whole food in its natural state, the more I could see with increasing clarity the inherent dysfunction in our culture. I realized that the literal geographical distance that had separated me from my food source in the past was a major contributing factor in my disordered eating.

Feeling good in my body, mind, and spirit was a freedom I had never felt before. Back when I was traveling around the world, I had begun to open up to others about my struggle with food, and I was amazed at how many others were experiencing this "secret" struggle with food as well—and were also afraid to talk about it because of the shame they felt. I saw the benefit people experienced when they did choose to talk about their struggle with food and weight more openly. This was when I first understood how many others suffered in silence, and that I was not alone.

Over time it became clear to me that I was meant to help others discover the same freedom I had discovered in the garden. This desire to help others inspired me to learn as much as possible about why we get hooked on the particular foods that keep us caught in the struggle and how we can make healthier food and lifestyle choices that free us from this struggle. This not only led me back to school to become a registered holistic nutritionist (RHN) but also inspired me to study yoga and meditation and become a certified yoga teacher. These unique paths of study allowed me to fuse Eastern and Western wisdom and knowledge into an integrated holistic approach to healthier living that I now have the privilege to share with others.

What's in the Craving?

It sounds so simple: eat when you're hungry and stop when you're full. You may feel frustrated at someone even trying to suggest that this is a simple concept, especially if you would describe yourself as a chronic overeater. Although I quite often point towards "overeaters" as people who struggle with food, they are definitely not the only ones. You don't even have to be overweight to fall into this category. Many people of *normal* weight who rarely overeat spend much of their lives in a continuous struggle with food and weight. We all know what it feels like to *crave* something, to feel the *urge* to eat, regardless of whether we're actually hungry or not. Why does this happen? Why do we overeat (or struggle with trying to prevent overeating), and why is it so difficult for so many to stop eating once they are full? What has changed to create such a rapid and dramatic increase in obesity rates in such a short amount of time? Have we collectively lost all willpower and self-control? Have *we* changed? No, we haven't changed, but our food supply has, and what we've come to accept as "normal" has shifted drastically.

If you repeatedly revert back to your old ingrained habits of overeating despite trying *everything* you possibly could, then the information provided in this book is going to help you step into a new level of self-awareness. Awareness is required for change to occur. Once you are aware of your habits, you can then consciously choose to change them.

Can We Be Addicted to Food?

I see clients on a daily basis who tell me they're hooked. Hooked? On what—cocaine, methamphetamines, alcohol . . . *heroin*? No, these clients profess that their lives are being taken over by their readily available, legal drug of choice: bagels, donuts, cheese, chips, ice cream, pizza, soda, and the list goes on. In other words: refined sugar, fat, salt, and processed foods. They're hooked; they can't stop thinking about food until they get their "fix," and this addiction is wreaking havoc on their lives.

Can we actually become *addicted* to a survival-based necessity like food? How do we distinguish between food addiction and our bodies telling us to eat? For many years, the medical community discredited the idea that there is such a thing as food addiction—until recently. Although it's still a highly debated topic, there has been a recent surge of research in this area, with many results pointing towards the similarities between food and drug addiction. Although an actual diagnosis of food addiction has not yet been defined within the medical community, food addiction researchers are noting a striking resemblance between food addiction and the diagnostic criteria for substance dependence.

These characteristics strike both a personal and now a professional chord. In my holistic nutrition consulting practice, my clients repeatedly describe these all-too-familiar addictive tendencies toward food. I've adapted the list of seven criteria for substance dependence from the *Diagnostic and Statistical Manual for Mental Disorders,* or the DSM IV-TR (APA, 2000) to demonstrate just how similar these addictions are:

1. **Increased tolerance to a substance.** Where once a single cupcake would do the trick, now you tend to reach for three or four to "satisfy" that craving. To get the desired effect you have to consume larger quantities; the same quantity of sugar (or fat, or salt) over time has a diminished effect, and an increasing amount of food is required to satisfy you.

2. **Substance is taken in larger amounts and for a longer period than the person originally intended.** You keep telling yourself that Monday you'll eat healthier, yet in this moment you can't seem to stop—a common symptom in people who struggle with food.

3. **Persistent desire or repeated unsuccessful attempts to quit or control use.** Think of the cycle of yo-yo dieting, with repeated attempts to exert willpower, only to regain the weight and return to the foods you know are keeping you hooked.

4. **Spending a great deal of time obtaining, using, or recovering from the substance.** Time is spent thinking about what, where, when, and how much to consume these addictive foods. Obsessing about what you should or shouldn't eat, or how much you weigh and how much you need to lose. Time may also be taken away from work or personal life to allow for recovery from a binge or from the harmful effects of food products.

5. **Important social, occupational, or recreational activities are given up or reduced.** You may avoid going out with friends because you're ashamed of what you look like or because you would rather stay home and eat (which may or may not turn into a binge).

6. **Use continues despite knowledge of adverse consequences.** This is when your food choices start to have a negative impact on your quality of

life. Perhaps you're unable to stop overeating, despite knowing that these addictive foods cause ill effects such as weight gain, mood swings, and decreased sex drive. Being overweight or obese can also have a negative impact on the quality of life, from expensive healthcare bills to increased risk of associated diseases, negative social stigma, reduced social contact, and reduced physical activity.

7. **Characteristic withdrawal symptoms**. When giving up your most addictive foods, you feel classic symptoms of withdrawal such as headaches, mood swings, lethargy, and depression.

It's not just the consumption of a substance that defines the addiction, as many people drink alcohol in their lifetime without ever becoming alcoholic. It's important to note that, like all addictions, we don't necessarily become addicted to the food (or wine, prescription drugs, reality television show, etc.) as such; people become addicted to the stimulation, the sedation, or other physical responses that these foods produce in them. Food addiction not only prompts behavioral changes, but also biological changes. As we will explore in chapter 3, whether someone is struggling with an addiction to cocaine or an addiction to processed foods, similar changes occur in the brain.

Food addiction is still a very new and complex field of study, but we don't need formal recognition by the medical community to know that in reality, millions of people are struggling with their relationship with food. People feel "hooked" on food just as others feel "hooked" on drugs. Whether you call it food addiction, disordered eating, compulsive overeating, uncontrollable cravings, or binge eating, people are struggling with food and are suffering as a result.

How Did This Happen?

Our values and culture have changed in such a way that, unlike our ancestors, most people no longer grow their own food and actually live far from where much of what we consume is actually grown. Given the sheer geographic distance that separates most of the population from their original food source, and considering what's being stocked on the shelves in grocery stores (highly processed, packaged foods), just about everyone has a dysfunctional relationship with food to some degree. I personally can't think of one person who is completely unaffected by this culturally pervasive issue; however, some people get "hooked" and struggle with it more than others. This doesn't mean that you have to grow your own garden to heal a disordered relationship with food, but it does require reconnecting to whole foods in some way that feels good for you, as we will explore throughout this book.

From a physiological perspective, our bodies haven't changed much for thousands of years, yet the food we eat has changed drastically in a very short amount of time. Going back to the initial question— can we be addicted to food?—Anne Katherine, MA, author of *Anatomy of a Food Addiction*, points to the answer. She defines the term "food addiction" as a "physical, biochemical condition of the body that creates cravings for refined carbohydrates, sugar, and fat."[1]

In the context of food addiction, the more important question is: can we be addicted to *real* food? I use this term "real" food as a loose term to describe whole foods in comparison to heavily processed foods. In my opinion, nature would not have played such a cruel joke as to hook us on mangoes, heavenly though they are. It's worth mentioning that there are, however, few situations where addiction is inherent in nature. Human breast milk—which is real food for babies—is an addictive substance by nature's design to strengthen the bond between a baby and mother. That aside, when it comes to food addiction, we aren't talking about real, whole foods, although we do repeatedly mistake these man-made "food-like" products for real food. As we will see, despite our built-in mechanisms that drive us to eat real food, "food-like" substances have hijacked our brain. Fake, processed foods make it very difficult to stop eating and drive us to eat more of them, regardless of hunger or fullness signals. It's what is causing so many people to spiral downward into cycles of food cravings, food addiction, mild disordered eating, and full-blown eating disorders.

Does This Sound Like You?

The development and maintenance of an unhealthy relationship with food can be a subtle process that's easily hidden not only from others but also from yourself. Typically overt symptoms, such as weight gain, depression, severe mood swings, or a diagnosis of heart disease or diabetes, are often the motivating factors that wake us up to our habitual patterns of eating and living.

In his research, author and former FDA commissioner David Kessler (*The End of Overeating*) wanted to estimate how many people have food addictive personalities. In Kessler's presentation at Authors@Google,[2] he shared three characteristics that are synonymous with food addiction. These characteristics are related to "hyper-palatable foods," a term used in the food industry to describe processed foods high in sugar, fat, and salt.

1. **Loss of control in the face of hyper-palatable food.** You have a difficult time resisting foods high in sugar, fat, and salt.
2. **Lack of satiation in the face of hyper-palatable food**. It takes longer to get the "I'm full" cue to stop eating.
3. **Preoccupation with hyper-palatable foods between meals**. This means that a large amount of your mental time and thought capacity goes toward food. You're thinking about what you're going to eat next while you're currently eating something, or you're at work and you're preoccupied with what you're going to eat for dinner, or you're eating dinner and you're thinking about dessert.

As mentioned, the overweight and obese are not the only ones struggling with these issues. Many people of so-called normal weight also suffer from preoccupation with weight and food. Based on his research, Kessler estimates the percentage of people who display food addictive characteristics to be:

- 50 percent of obese individuals
- 30 percent of overweight individuals
- 17 percent of lean individuals

Kessler also estimates that these statistics translate to roughly 70 million people in the United States alone who are struggling with some level of food addictive characteristics.

If you're asking yourself, "Am I struggling with an addiction to food?" take a moment to jump to Appendix A and fill out the Yale Food Addiction Scale, developed by Ashley Gearhardt of Yale University. This is a quick and easy way to know if your struggle with food is actually a food-addiction.

You've heard it before: the first step is admitting you have a problem. Chances are, if you're reading this book, you already know you struggle with food to some extent. If you resonate with Kessler's three characteristics of food addiction or the questions presented in the Yale Food Addiction Scale, you're not alone. If you've been beating yourself up for being this way, this book will help you take the steps you need to free yourself—with self-compassion and loving-kindness— from this struggle.

Don't Fight the Elephant: Ending the Struggle

Our collective dysfunctional relationship with food is causing us much pain and suffering. As I have discovered, food can be such an incredible source of pleasure in our lives, but for many, it is more often a source of struggle, pain, and hardship. Imagine yourself standing outside in a vast open field under a big blue sky. Now imagine standing in front of a big, beautiful elephant. Looking at this elephant with curiosity, wonder, and awe can be an incredible experience. You can touch, feel, and smell its skin, listen to its unique sounds, and perhaps sit on the elephant and be carried on a journey to incredible places. But as soon as you try to control it or wrestle with it, you're going to struggle— and you're going to lose.

This is a good metaphor for our struggle with food. It can be a doorway into a new way of seeing the world, a doorway into delight, pleasure, and freedom. Or it can be one of the most challenging experiences of your life, and once you gain awareness and understanding, it's largely your choice. You don't need to try and fight the elephant anymore; you can simply appreciate it for what it is.

The Six "Hooks" of Overeating

Eating copious amounts of food until we feel uncomfortably full is illogical, yet we do it anyway. It's irrational, yet many stay trapped in this cycle. Why do so many people do this to themselves?

I spent years studying why people struggle with food addictions, why people overeat, and why millions of people waste years of their precious lives worrying about how much they weigh, and what they should or shouldn't do about it.

I looked to the sciences as I studied holistic nutrition and the Eastern wisdom traditions as I studied yoga and meditation. I looked to nature, food, plants, other professionals, mentors and spiritual teachers, clients, friends and family, random strangers I observed eating, books and textbooks, websites and blogs, and of course my own experience. All in search of why so many people want to end their battle with food—but haven't yet been able to.

Over the years of studying this issue, what I discovered was that there are many different factors involved in our collective food struggle. All of these factors can essentially be grouped into six interconnected, somewhat overlapping categories that

I call "hooks," because they keep people hooked on their struggle with food. These hooks are environmental, physiological, behavioral, mental, emotional, and spiritual.

The information I learned about each of these six hooks was nothing less than shocking and forced a radical shift in perspective, a necessary shift that provided an opportunity to question my belief systems and step into a new way of living and being. I invite you to approach this book with the same level of openness. As my mother says, "take the best and leave the rest." I'm not asking you to take anything I've written in this book at face value. Explore the ideas presented and, by all means, experiment! Carve out a path that *feels good* and resonates for you. I completely recognize and accept that what might be true for one person may not be for another, especially when it comes to food and how we relate to it—a touchy subject indeed. What I do encourage, however, is to open yourself up to the *possibility* that this book may contain some nuggets of wisdom that may improve your relationship with food and end your food-related suffering. As Albert Einstein said, "We can't solve problems by using the same kind of thinking we used when we created them." Indeed, this book is about so much more than just food; it encompasses a holistic, multidimensional approach to breaking free from your struggle with food and living a more joyful life.

Imagine that each of these six hooks—environmental, physiological, behavioral, mental, emotional, and spiritual—represents a string on a guitar. When a guitar is perfectly tuned and each string is in resonance with the other strings, it makes beautiful sounds of musical harmony. It feels aligned and in sync. This is when we are completely unhooked and free from the struggle. If just one string is out of tune, it will still make music, but with a discordant sound that is slightly off and out of tune. Now imagine the unpleasant sound the guitar would make if every string was out of tune. When this happens in our own lives, we get disharmonious living, and what manifests are symptoms like weight gain, depression, lack of motivation, mood swings, and *dis-ease*. These symptoms are simply intuitive messages that your body communicates to let you know that you need to tune the string(s) on your guitar so you can resonate in harmony and, in turn, radiate that frequency to the rest of the world.

How to Use This Book

You can learn how to unhook yourself from each hook, so that you can function optimally as a fully integrated human being. This book is divided into six parts:

1. Environmental
2. Physiological
3. Behavioral
4. Mental
5. Emotional
6. Spiritual

Each part is broken down into two chapters: Hooked and Unhooked. In the Hooked chapters, you will learn why you get hooked on your struggle with food from this particular perspective, and in the Unhooked chapters, I offer you suggestions on how to free yourself from the struggle. In addition to the practical advice and many tips you will read throughout this book. I offer specific exercises that you can implement immediately to help unhook yourself from your food struggle. I also invite you to take time to "pause and reflect," an opportunity for you to put down the book, turn your attention inward, and explore your relationship with food. You will also see text boxes with specific, relevant quotes from my favorite authors sprinkled throughout the text to help you gain deeper insight into the presented topic. I suggest that you dedicate a journal or blank workbook that you can use in conjunction with reading this book, jotting down thoughts, insights, and answers to the questions presented in each of the chapters.

Not Another Diet

I believe there are many of you, like me, who have tried many different weight-loss methods, diet plans, exercise regimens, and fasting protocols, and eventually found yourself right back where you started, overcome by feelings of hopelessness and despair. If you are experiencing food addiction, chronic overeating, obsessive thoughts about weight, food, and body image, constantly agonizing about what to eat or what not to eat or how to avoid the craving and binging, or simply are lost and confused about the steps to take to lead you to a healthier you—then I encourage you to keep reading. This is not another diet book. If your life is a constant struggle with food and you are still searching for answers, I hope this book will open a window into your life and allow a ray of hope. May it light your path and guide you towards a healthier and happier lifestyle.

Implementing these sound principles will help you on your journey to freedom—freedom from the fixation on food, obsessive weight control, and living with the burden of fear and emotional uncertainty. The road ahead can be a healthy, vibrant lifestyle, full of unlimited possibilities, and a deep knowing that you are a divine miracle, here to fulfill your highest purpose on this journey we call life.

It *is* possible to have a relationship with food that feels normal, that feels less crazy and compulsive and more comfortable, that feels sane and, yes, even *joyful*. It *is* possible to have a relationship with food that brings you happiness, pleasure, confidence, a sense of connection, and vibrant health. These are all within your reach. Actually, it would be better to think of it not as something within your reach *out there*, separate from you, but as a reality that is already *here*, waiting for you to remember and align with it.

This book is a result of my desire to help others achieve long-lasting health and reconnect to a joyful life, especially for those who are willing to try something that may seem radically new, yet so profoundly simple, to heal their relationship with food and their body. My intention is to give you hope that you too can move past your preoccupation with food. It is not my intention to try to radicalize your lifestyle, but rather to share with you my experiences and insights into how you too can achieve vibrant health and happiness.

I hope that the solutions in this book can be of great benefit to you on your journey to health. My deepest wish is that you experience true joy and freedom from struggle and become inspired to live the life you have always dreamed of.

"The time is now for transformation. It is a new era and we are poised with the opportunity to bring in a new consciousness, and co-create a new reality. Why? Because the light within each of us has been turned on, and it's our job to turn that light on brighter and brighter until all false thought forms dissolve in the light of our Truth."

—Dr. Michelle L. Casto

PART ONE

The Environmental Hook

"It is no measure of health to be well adjusted to a profoundly sick society."

—Jiddu Krishnamurti

Chapter 1

How Our Environment Hooks Us

Now, more than ever, information is being shared about how our global food environment is contributing to our compulsion to keep eating, and processed, food-like substances are taking center stage. What wrong turn did we take to find ourselves in a place where we now have to educate ourselves about the difference between edible "fabricated" food and wholesome real food; where the price of these processed foods has become incredibly cheap, yet our healthcare costs as a nation have skyrocketed; where more people are obese, yet paradoxically are "dieting" more than ever before? Part of the challenge is that our food environment has changed so drastically in such a short period of time that we now have to navigate through an increasingly confusing food situation. How did all this happen? In order to move in the right direction, we need to understand where we are now and how we got here.

Tightly Held Beliefs

Beliefs are opinions that we accept as being true for us—and we all have our share, especially when it comes to food. Our beliefs about food tend to carry a heavy emotional charge. I don't think anything can rouse people into heated debate like nutrition can—except for maybe religion or politics. Countless times I've witnessed

3

people go into panic or rage mode when defending their personal beliefs about food, such as defending the rights of animals and advocating veganism, or arguing that it's impossible to be healthy without eating meat.

Everyone wants validation; we want to be right and don't want to hear or be told that the beliefs that guide our behavior are not always grounded in truth. Some of our beliefs are deeply entrenched, especially those that define us as individuals, including the way we eat. When we put ourselves in a definitive "dietary box," adding concrete labels to our dietary patterns (whether you define yourself as a "meat eater" or "vegan"), these beliefs can be static and inflexible, and lead to rigid ways of thinking. When we label and rigidly define our food philosophy and belief systems (BS), we leave less room for new information to filter through, moving us away from our inherent wisdom and becoming more wrapped up in the ensuing debate about who's right and who's wrong.

So much of the way we eat is due to deeply engrained beliefs that historically have been created by the agricultural industries and food companies, perpetuated by lobbyists and backed by government. Many of these food-related beliefs have been with us since before the 1950s, and it is difficult to remember a time when we all lived closely connected to the abundant earth and ate whole foods.

Pause & Reflect: Your Beliefs, Up Close and Personal

Take a moment to pause and reflect on what your belief systems are regarding food. Do you believe that you need to consume milk for calcium? Do you believe that you need to consume animal flesh to grow your muscles big and strong? Do you believe carbohydrates are bad? Do you believe you need to eat tofu to be a healthy vegetarian? Do you think that grains should be a part of a healthy diet? Do you believe that all sugar is evil? Do you believe that the only way for you to lose weight is through depriving yourself on a diet? Do you believe that "heart healthy" oils like olive oil are good for you? Do you believe that consuming salt prevents dehydration?

Many of these traditional beliefs helped shape the way we think about food, but do these convictions hold up under closer scrutiny? We all need to put our assumptions about food under a magnifying glass. What are some of your major food-related beliefs? What caused you to have these beliefs? Where did they come from? Was it something taught in school? Did a commercial inform you of this, a magazine article, or perhaps a family member? Is it possible that some of your beliefs about food might not be serving your best interest? Are you willing to explore what's actually true for you and your body, apart from what you believe is true?

When a Tomato Is No Longer a Tomato

Today, when it comes to food, everything has changed. We're forced to navigate an increasingly complex food environment with extreme caution. We can no longer say the word "tomato" and agree about what this means, even if they appear (somewhat) similar on the outside. A tomato genetically modified to be perfectly round with thick skin and a waxy coat when picked green weeks prior to ripening and gassed with ripening chemicals when it arrives at its destination is worlds apart from the organic purple heirloom tomato that I picked ripe off the vine this morning. These tomatoes are not the same—right down to their molecular makeup. Although we call them both tomatoes, we now have to learn to decipher between the two. In some regards, I consider the first to be somewhat "fake"—a man-made food product and a result of our current food industry. This is the food environment that most of us now live in. The second example is what I loosely call "real" food—a result of collaborating with the natural ways of nature. I say "loosely call 'real' food" because of course there's no exact cut-and-dry definition of "real" versus "fake" food, but rather general descriptors we can apply. See the section Whole Food Versus Processed Food later in this chapter for a more thorough description.

Genetically modified foods are one example, yet we also need to recognize what has become our socially acceptable definition of food. Author and food journalist Michael Pollan pointed this out when he popularized the phrase "food-like substance." He suggests that just because you can put it in your mouth and it may taste good doesn't make it real food. This way of perceiving these processed and packaged "foods" has become an accepted belief system in our culture, much to our detriment. What led us down the brightly colored aisles upon aisles of packaged foods that have an infinite shelf life and clever marketing schemes, where Convenience with a capital "C" dominates the marketplace—at all costs?

Scientific Reductionism

In the sixteenth and seventeenth centuries, major scientific discoveries had long-lasting and far-reaching consequences, fundamentally changing the way we look at the world. While many were beneficial, unfortunately some had negative implications for our current food environment.

René Descartes popularized the method of analytic thinking, or breaking up complex phenomena into pieces to understand the behaviors of the whole from the properties of its parts.[3] It was during this time that the mechanistic view took hold—essentially relating the miracles of life to the clockworks of a machine, and thus "mechanistic thinking" was born. This worldview still predominates our perceptions despite incredible discoveries in quantum physics—discoveries that show how our thoughts influence matter—the interconnection of our mind and body—and that we are indeed made up of more than the sum of our parts.

Rooted within this paradigm of the mechanistic model, chemist Antoine-Laurent Lavoisier (1743–1794) defined the calorie, a measure of the energy in food, thus equating food to fuel to feed the "machine." Then, in the nineteenth century, an English doctor and chemist named William Prout isolated and identified carbohydrates, proteins, and fats, what are now known as macronutrients. One by one, new vitamins and minerals were identified in food, and step-by-step we lost greater sight of the whole—the greater meaning in whole food—in favor of a reductionist mentality limiting our view of food to mere numbers and nutrients.

As a result, we now tend to look at food with a "microscopic view," only able to see one isolated part of the whole at a time, when in fact it would be more appropriate to look at food through a kaleidoscope, in which all the beautiful colors and integrated components mesh into each other and are inexorably linked together.

Driven by the media, the food industry, and government agencies, the dialogue then became all about which nutrients were "good" and which were "bad," and before we knew it we were looking to experts for nutritional advice to help steer our eating habits in the "right" direction—only to seduce us further and further away from the miracle of *real* food.

"Since nutrients, as compared with foods, are invisible and therefore slightly mysterious, it falls to the scientists (and to the journalists through whom the scientists speak) to explain the hidden reality of foods to us. To enter a world in which you dine on unseen nutrients, you need lots of expert help."

—Michael Pollan

In his book *The Web of Life*, Fritjof Capra talks about "systems thinking," describing things in terms of *connectedness, relationships,* and *context,* as opposed to "mechanist thinking." He states: "According to the systems view, the essential properties of an organism, or living system, are properties of the whole, which none of the parts have. They arise from the interactions and relationships among the parts. These properties are destroyed when the system is dissected . . . into isolated elements."[4] Essentially, we can't isolate individual nutrients from the miracle of the interconnected perfection of the whole food from which the nutrient came and still call it the same thing with the same benefits.

A perfect example of trying to isolate a single nutrient from the whole food from which it emanated is the famous Cancer Prevention Study of 1995. After discovering the health benefits of beta-carotene in carrots, two studies were conducted to try to prove the health benefits of this nutrient for cancer patients. The participants were given these micronutrients in isolation, not within the whole foods in which they are normally found. To the researchers' surprise, they found that isolated beta-carotene supplementation is associated with significantly higher incidence of lung cancer and mortality, and the trial had to be abandoned.[5]

Despite all the information we are inundated with about nutrition, most of it contradictory, science actually doesn't have the definitive answers to our diet woes that we are searching for. As Michal Pollan states in *Food Rules,* " . . . in fact science knows a lot less about nutrition than you would expect—that in fact nutrition science is, to put it charitably, a very *young* science." It's still not completely definitive what goes on inside our bodies when we eat chocolate or munch on a piece of celery. They can see trends and correlations, but relatively speaking, they're only scratching the tip of the iceberg.

It's impossible for us to fully grasp the manner in which one tiny nutrient like beta-carotene works in relation to the synergistic magic of the whole carrot. There are an untold number of properties working together in carrots that lend this root vegetable its health-promoting and life-giving force, properties we may never be able to fully comprehend—as doing so would be to know the mystery and secrets of life itself. This reductionist approach, now solely driven by profit, ultimately led to the wave of processed food-like substances masquerading as real food.

I'm certainly not saying that all the incredible discoveries of individual nutrients aren't beneficial. All discoveries are important. However, when we look at isolated nutrients (through the microscope) and not the greater whole (kaleidoscope), we lose the connection to the deeper meaning and miracle of real food. This predominant worldview is one that separates us from nature, quite literally, as seen by the large geographic distance that separates most people from their food source. We're out of touch with ourselves and with nature, and this disconnect amplifies competition within a trillion-dollar food industry, vying for our food dollars.

> "Nutrition arguments are almost invariably about single nutrients taken out of their context, single foods taken out of their dietary context, or single risk factors and diseases taken out of their lifestyle context. Single-nutrient arguments are 'reductive' in that they reduce diets and food choices to one simple decision: eat this or avoid that, and all problems will be solved. Food companies love this approach because they can use it to say that their particular products have special health benefits. But few issues in nutrition are that simple."
>
> —Marion Nestle, *What to Eat*

Whole Food Versus Processed Food

Whole food is food that comes directly from the earth, (from nature) without any—or very minimal—processing or man-made interference.

> "Whole food (noun): food that has been processed or refined as little as possible and is free from additives or other artificial substances."
>
> —Oxford Dictionary

Whole foods are what I tend to refer to as "real" foods. When I picked berries right off the bush this morning, I was reminded of how fresh, whole, and delicious real food is. Despite food science continuously trying to outsmart nature, there is no amount of science that can do a better job of replicating these berries that are already "designed" to perfection.

Whole foods start to lose their full "wholeness" when we process and even cook them. When we cook foods we start to change the chemical composition of the food, further losing and destroying vitamins, minerals, enzymes, and phytonutrients—just to name a few. Depending on the method of cooking, the length of time, and the temperatures the food is subjected to, foods can be drastically altered from their original state. When we cook food, we also lose a large portion of its inherent water content.

It is my personal opinion that on a cellular level, our infinitely intelligent bodies recognize real, whole foods as optimal—as what we are anatomically and physiologically designed to consume. And to a certain extent, when nutrients are lost from our food in the refinement (and even cooking) process, whether it's vitamins, water, or any other nutrient, our body has to work harder to compensate in some way to make up for the loss, either by depleting its nutritional reserves or by simply doing the best it can with the "incomplete" nutritional resource available, compromising its function. Water is a perfect example of this. When we cook food, we remove much of its water content—that's why cooked foods can be dehydrating. I immediately notice how dehydrated I become after eating a cooked meal. It's ironic that we then add layers upon layers to the dysfunction by recommending the population supports their chronic dehydration not by correcting the underlying imbalance—eating whole foods—but by drinking no less than eight cups of water a day!

"The natural world is what our bodies recognize as safe and supportive, thus causing maintenance and replication of cells. Our bodies do not recognize processed foods; therefore, they have to work harder to digest and assimilate any minor nutrients that may be derived from such food. Stress is not just the fight or flight reaction that produces adrenaline, it is also the added hard work of digesting, filtering, pumping, eliminating, and integrating what is perceived as foreign to our systems."

—Pam Montgomery, *Plant Spirit Healing*

The heavy processing of refined, fragmented foods, and all the nutrients lost in those foods due to these industrial processes, is only part of the equation that makes up what I refer to as "fake" foods. The second part of the equation is what is then added back after so many vital nutrients are stripped away. Added to the mix are thousands upon thousands of other "ingredients" that are not found in nature but are chemically fabricated in a production plant to help the food achieve its most desirable taste, texture, smell, shelf life, and other marketable qualities. The real problem is that these packaged fake foods are what most people have come to accept as "normal," when they are anything but normal. They make berry flavoring without real berries and vanilla flavoring without real vanilla bean. Do we really know the long-term consequences of eating these imitation foods? And can this honestly be better than the real thing? Maybe only better monetarily—and only for the very few people reaping the profits.

In his book *Salt Sugar Fat*, Michael Moss describes the Kool-Aid brand managers' efforts to market one of their "imitation" food products:

> The Kool Bursts were engineered to evoke the image of fresh fruit in as many ways as possible: They were made in a variety of imitation fruit flavors, including cherry, grape, orange, and tropical punch, and they were given the most enticing imitation aromas that lab technicians could devise so that when the bottles were opened, they emitted powerful fruity smells. Even the bottles promulgated the mythology of health . . . .[6]

Despite the "healthy" advertising marketed directly to children, this brightly colored drink is surprisingly sweeter than Coke, and at one point was stirring up close to 600 million gallons a year.[7] This disconnect from nature is what defines our current food environment and redefines the very basis of our relationship with food—to real, living food that comes from the earth. Instead we're living in a society with many children who don't even know what a cucumber plant looks like or how tomatoes grow, or that chips and French fries are made from potatoes.

This really hit home for me one day when my friend's little brother was drinking a freshly opened, sweet Thai coconut (an incredible, hydrating gift from nature) and exclaimed: "Man, I wish they would make something that tastes this good!" I looked at him with a bewildered look on my face as I grasped the magnitude of what he actually just said and replied: "*They* already did; you're holding it in your hand." I knew he meant he wished that the food industry could make a drink with coconut flavoring that could come in a colorful can and that he could easily buy whenever he wanted it, which, not surprisingly, they recently have. This thought process not only reflects how disconnected we can become from our food source, but also how we, as a culture, drive consumer demand for the very same products that further perpetuate our separation from nature.

"It is as if we are banging our head against the wall. When we stop, we discover our headache is gone and it is easier to meditate. Meanwhile, modern technology is studying the physiology of how to live normally while banging our head against the wall. Because most people are

normally banging their head against the wall, we are considered abnormal because we choose to stop."

—**Gabriel Cousens**, *Spiritual Nutrition*

Of course, there is a largely grey, undefined area that lies in the middle of the polar ends of "real" whole foods versus "fake" processed foods. Raising these questions as to what we define as real food is a good place to start and encourages us to question what we're eating. Ultimately it's up to you to use your intuition and common sense to determine what you define as real or fake food and to ask yourself if the way you're eating is connecting you to—or separating you from—the natural ways of nature. I came to realize that what we've collectively agreed on as "normal" is a far cry from normal. The fact that millions of people eat these foods and continue to live with excess weight and disease is not proof of the safety of these processed foods, but rather a testament to the miracle of the human body and the abuse that it can endure.

The Birth of Fragmented Foods

The "food-as-nutrient" concept became popular during the industrial food revolution with the birth of refined foods. Whole foods were starting to be dissected, separated, and processed, and the food industry used new nutritional terminology to rationalize these "food-like products" and make scientific sense to the public about the new food environment they (food companies, government, and agricultural big business) had fabricated and now tried to control. Fake foods flooded the markets and only reinforced the food-as-nutrient mentality. Whatever key nutrient was currently deemed "good" by mainstream media was "in": "Fortified with Vitamin C," "High in Fiber," "Source of Omega-3s." And whatever nutrient was out of favor was deemed "bad," which companies also used to sell their fake-food products: "Low in Saturated Fats" and "Gluten Free!"

"The trouble with the whole notion of 'evil' and 'blessed' ingredients is that they help the food industry sell us processed foods that are free of the evil thing or full of the blessed one. We buy them, not realizing they may contain many other ingredients that aren't good for us."

—**Michael Pollan**

So many singular nutrients have passed both in and out of vogue, leaving the consumer more and more confused, entrenching a good/bad, all-or-nothing mentality that keeps millions of people walking a dietary tightrope. As one client said to me, "The contradictory overlap of all the different diets I've been on has left me unable to eat anything at all, as all foods have been vilified and deemed 'bad' in at least one diet I've been on."

When you walk into the grocery store, pick up a package, and read the food label, this is an example of reductionist thinking within the framework of the industrial food complex. We wouldn't need food labels if we were still eating whole foods, would we? Apples, bananas, peaches, cucumbers, lettuce, broccoli—*whole foods*— don't need a label. (I do, however, recommend that if you are going to buy packaged food that you do read the label. This point is raised to illustrate the concept of packaged "fabricated" foods versus whole foods not requiring any such packaging.) But over time, the industry has led us to believe that the food they are fabricating is still real food. This compartmentalized approach to food is indeed what's developed into the standard American diet (SAD) and has led not only to a plethora of fake foods lining the grocery shelves, but health epidemics like heart disease, diabetes, cancer, and obesity running rampant and a healthcare bill that has skyrocketed along with it. Ironically, this reductionist thinking is evident when you visit your local health food store and you see row upon row of supplements and health "products" touting the benefits of individual nutrients. All sides of the equation are using these methods to sell us products—not food, but *products*.

When you think of it logically, does it make sense to take a whole food, strip it of most of its nutrients, refine it down to a single nutrient, and sell it as a supplement, instead of just eating the whole food that has everything inherent in it that our bodies recognize as optimally nourishing?*

We've gone from having a direct experience with nature, our *original* food source, to approaching our meals with analytical minds, reducing food to calories, numbers, and nutrients, a mindset deeply rooted in what I call nutritional BS—those belief systems handed down to us for several generations from government and the food and agriculture industries. This has created the perception of food and nutrition as a massive, convoluted, and complicated topic, engrained within a set of shared yet unexamined assumptions and belief systems.

---

* There are certain situations where supplementation can be beneficial, but generally we don't all need to be taking large amounts of supplements on a daily basis. Please consult with a Doctor or Holistic Health Practitioner before taking any supplements.

Mindless Eating

Up to this point, we've looked at the greater cultural context that has shaped and defined our food environment, including key events in history—like the industrial food revolution—that have led us to this point where we are surrounded by processed foods, fast food restaurants, and accepted cultural norms that have largely influenced our eating habits. Now let's narrow our focus and look at our more immediate eating environment.

Not surprisingly, the surroundings we find ourselves in can dramatically influence a person's food intake.[8] As we will explore throughout this book, and as I'm sure you already know, the urge or desire to eat or overeat often has nothing to do with hunger. These external, environmental factors not only influence what we eat, but also how much we eat and when we choose to stop. Our direct environment affects how we monitor our consumption of food and what consumption level we perceive as normal. The bad news is that even though these environmental cues are ubiquitous, most people aren't even aware they're being influenced by them.

Brian Wansink, PhD, director of the Cornell Food and Brand Lab at Cornell University, has conducted hundreds of food experiments looking at environmental cues that trigger people to overeat. He shares many of the findings in his book *Mindless Eating: Why We Eat More Than We Think*. If you haven't read this book, I highly recommend that you do. What you will find is nothing short of shocking.

According to Wansink, influential environmental factors can be organized into two main categories:[9] the eating environment and the food environment.

The Eating Environment

1. **The eating atmosphere.** Restaurant owners know it's all about the ambiance. The music that is played as well as the lighting in a restaurant can and does affect how much people eat. That's why places like McDonald's create a hectic atmosphere to get people in and out—fast—while other restaurants play relaxing music to encourage people to sit, stay, and drink more expensive wine.

2. **The eating effort.** The food that is most readily available and convenient to eat is the food you are most likely to go for. Increased effort to obtain food results in decreased consumption. With fast food readily available on every corner and food now available at any time of day, it's more challenging (but not impossible) to steer clear of these packaged, processed foods.

3. **Eating with others.** Would you be surprised if I told you that other people influence how much you eat? It's true: how we eat is highly influenced by those around us.[10] People mimic the intake level of those around them, adjusting upwards or downwards based on how much those people around them choose to eat.[11] The amount of food we eat also tends to increase as the number of eating companions increases.[12] This is because when we look to those around us, we adopt a belief system about what is acceptable or reasonable. One very strong social cue that usually goes unnoticed is continuing to eat until everyone else has finished eating, because it is regarded as socially acceptable to keep eating as long as others are doing the same, whether you are still feeling hungry or not.

4. **Eating distractions.** We live in a culture that associates eating with every single event, activity, and time of day, as well as a culture that promotes eating on the go. Did you know that roughly 20 percent of food is eaten in the car? If you tend to eat while being preoccupied with other activities like watching TV, checking e-mail, or talking on the phone, chances are you'll eat more without even realizing it. More on mindful eating in chapter 8.

"[Food companies] were already trying to sell their products in an environment in which there were twice as many calories as anybody needed. Now, they had to grow their profits every ninety days. The result was that food companies had to seek new ways to market their foods. And they did that by making larger portions, by making food available absolutely everywhere, by making food as convenient as it could be, and by creating a social environment in which it was okay to eat all day long, in more places, in larger portions."

—Marion Nestle

The Food Environment

1. **Salience.** According to the Oxford Dictionary, salience is defined as something that is "most noticeable or important." Because food is everywhere, simply seeing or smelling a food can trigger unintentional eating. Unfortunately, if you tend to struggle with food, these sensory triggers will make food the "most noticeable" and prominent sensory stimuli within your environment, constantly reminding you to pay attention to something you'd rather not be distracted by. Our senses are what causes this salience effect to take place:

a. **Visibility**. Visibility can influence eating in two main ways. If we see food, there's more chance that we'll consume it, such as the sight of someone eating a donut, the sight of a bowl of M&Ms, food advertising, cooking shows, etc. The visual cue can be subtle yet powerful. In one study, when 30 Hershey's Kisses were placed on the desks of administrative assistants, the candies placed in clear jars were consumed 46 percent more quickly than those placed in opaque jars.[13] We're also cued by the sight of food already on our plates and tend to keep eating as long as there is food remaining. In another study,[14] Dr. Wansink created a "bottomless soup bowl" where tomato soup was imperceptibly refilled through concealed tubing that ran through the table and into the bottoms of the bowls. People eating from these "bottomless" bowls consumed 73 percent more soup (113 more calories) than those eating from normal bowls, but estimated that they ate only 4.8 calories more.

b. **Auditory cues.** These include the crinkling sound of someone opening up a bag of chips, food sizzling on the barbeque, someone describing their meal to you, or hearing an advertisement describe a food.

c. **Olfactory cues.** These include the smell of fresh-baked cookies, or the smell of food roasting in the oven.

d. **Taste.** The taste of specific combinations of foods (such as sugar, fat, and salt) can encourage us to keep eating.

2. **Variety.** Increased variety (even if it's only perceived) in the food supply will increase consumption and may contribute to the development and maintenance of obesity. Animal and human studies show that food consumption increases when there is more variety in a meal or diet, and that greater dietary variety is associated with increase in body weight and fat.[15] In one study,[16] researchers found that consumers ate 23 percent more yogurt when offered three flavors instead of just one. Given the abundance of food we see, with thousands upon thousands of packaged foods lining the shelves (there are about forty thousand products being sold in an average grocery store), this diversity is somewhat of an illusion. Consumers think they have unlimited food choices, but in reality, most of the choice is only a choice of packaging. There are actually very few plants required to make these processed foods, and in our era, corn, wheat, and soy predominate. Food

scientists have created thousands of derivatives from these three plants that show up on food labels disguised under a myriad of names. Most of these thousands of processed products are simply a combination of corn, wheat, and/or soy, plus sugar, fat, and salt, plus an added host of chemicals to lend the food a more stable "shelf life."

3. **Package and portion sizes.** Bigger packages mean more consumption, and now we have larger plates and portion sizes than ever before. Through various studies that Dr. Wansink has conducted, the results are consistent: people tend to eat about 20–30 percent more from larger packages compared to smaller packages, regardless of whether people are of normal weight or overweight. Despite the size of our dishes, we tend to fill them up and eat until we finish what's on our plates.

4. **Stockpiling.** If you try to save on your grocery bill by shopping at Costco, buying huge multipack, bulk-food items, you're likely to consume more of these foods. This is partly because they are more prominent and visible in the household, and as we previously witnessed, eating from larger packages encourages higher consumption of food.

5. **Size of serving container.** Wide or large food containers create consumption illusion. This is such a powerful cue that, even if the food doesn't taste good, most people will still eat more if they are eating from a bigger package. In another study that Dr. Wansink conducted, moviegoers were randomly given a medium (120 grams) or large (240 grams) container of free popcorn that was either fresh or stale (14 days old). They measured how much people ate after the movie ended, as well as viewers' perceived taste. Dr. Wansink explains: "We found that moviegoers who were given fresh popcorn ate 45.3 percent more popcorn when it was given to them in large containers. This container-size influence is so powerful that when the popcorn was disliked (in the case of the stale, 14-day-old popcorn), people still ate 33.6 percent more popcorn when eating from a large container than a medium-size container."[17]

Other cues can include:

1. **Emotional cues.** Many people are all too familiar with eating for comfort. We may be prompted to overeat when uncomfortable feelings of loneliness, anger, and sadness overcome us. More about emotional eating in chapter 9.

2. **Thoughts**. Thoughts of past or future events that make us anxious or nervous, or simply thoughts of specific foods or times we shared a special meal at a particular restaurant can cue us to eat.

3. **Time of day.** Research shows that overweight people are more influenced to eat by the time of day than normal-weight people. In one study, when researchers changed the clock, the overweight group ate more because they thought it was dinnertime, when it was actually still the afternoon.[7]

4. **Weather.** Food choices are often influenced by the weather: ever notice yourself crave soup on a rainy day?

Pause & Reflect: What Triggers You?

It's important to start identifying what cues you to eat, especially when you're not actually hungry. This will help you become more aware of what's driving your hunger. Awareness is key here; if you pay attention to what is triggering you to eat, you can start to work with these triggers in a gentle, mindful, and loving way.

What are some of the cues that trigger a craving, where thoughts of food hijack your mind? Is it a distinct social situation or particular location? Notice what distractions you preoccupy yourself with when you eat, like your phone or the TV. Notice the sights, smells, or sounds of food that can trigger you to eat. Notice if the time of day influences you to eat, despite not actually being hungry. Do specific thoughts trigger you? What about portion sizes? Start to notice all the details surrounding your relationship with food. These are just some of the many ways that you may be influenced to eat—no hunger required. The more you practice becoming aware of your triggers, over time you will gain deeper insight into what triggers you to eat. And as you will discover for yourself, awareness equates to choice.

How We Get Hooked

All the thousands of cues that take place in our environment act as powerful triggers that create an impulse motivating us to pursue the food of our desire. Once we are triggered by a cue, we get hooked, it grabs our full attention, and our minds get consumed with thoughts of wanting that food, stimulating a certain degree of excitement in us. And if we've had the sensory pleasure of indulgence in the past, this experience is also locked into our memory, making the arousal that much more intense.

The true power that food has over us is our *expectation* of the reward that we will receive from the food once it is eaten. This comes from our natural ability to *anticipate* the pleasure we will receive from it; this is what drives our desire. Have you ever craved a food for a few hours or even days, finally give in to the craving, and realize that it didn't taste as good as you imagined? Cravings consume our minds, locking our thoughts into repetitive thinking about whatever it is we crave, until we either satisfy the craving, or move on and focus on something else.

For many people, once they are triggered and food grabs their attention, an inner dialogue takes over:

"Man, that looks good, I would love to have some of that right now . . . "

"But it's high in fat, and you're trying to go on a diet, so you really shouldn't have it . . . "

"But I want it . . . "

"Well, you could always start your diet in the morning and eat this as your last indulgence . . . "

And on and on it goes like a ping-pong match, the all-consuming preoccupation with food. As soon as we start engaging in it, we actually amplify it. (As psychologists now know, trying to suppress thoughts can be remarkably counterproductive. If I tell you not to think about a white bear, what's the first thing that pops into your mind?) It then becomes more and more difficult to look away and get out of the cycle. The more we focus on whether we should or shouldn't eat something, the likelier it is that we are going to eat it. A slippery slope, indeed.

For many, this slippery slope feels like a downward spiral, and as a result people are searching with a fierce determination for guidance to help them make sense out of the chaos. Thus the booming of another billion-dollar industry that claims to have all the fast, easy, and effortless answers to end all your struggles—but only if you sign on the dotted line.

"The dieting industry is the only business in the world that has a 98 percent failure rate."

—Eating Disorder Foundation

The Diet Industry: Your Failure Equals Their Success

Talking about our food environment wouldn't be complete without addressing the other elephant in the room (next to the food companies dishing out their fake foods). The diet industry permeates our cultural perceptions of how we should relate to food and our bodies and is negatively affecting the well-being of millions of people.

"Diet" is one of the most highly misused and abused words in our culture today. I'm no gambler, but I'd be willing to bet the majority of people reading this book have misused this word in some way, with the most common form of expression being, "That's it; I'm going on a *diet!* (Starting on Monday, after I finish eating this last donut . . .)"

Today the word "diet" is strictly associated with weight loss, but it was not meant to mean a two-week hiatus to lose as much weight as possible in the shortest amount of time as possible—only to gain it right back. Today's concept of "diet" is restrictive and obviously unsustainable. We're using this dreaded D-word to describe a very stressful, self-consuming, restrictive behavior with food to achieve a goal that doesn't last and maybe doesn't even work at all—what a terrible paradigm to endure!

Pause & Reflect: What Is Your Relationship with Dieting?

Take a moment to reflect on how you relate to the concept of "dieting." What does the word "diet" mean to you? Do you typically eat one way most of the time and then drastically alter what you eat when you want to lose weight? Are you constantly trying the latest fad diet? How many different diets have you been on? How many of them actually worked for you? How many "lose 7 pounds in 7 days" programs have you tried? What about colonics, the Master Cleanse, the Atkins Diet, Jenny Craig, or Weight Watchers? If you lost some weight on a diet, only to regain it back (with a few extra pounds for good measure), then you're in the same boat as almost everyone else who's embarked on a new dieting regimen. The odds are stacked against the majority; 95 percent of all dieters regain their weight back in one to three years.

If you alter your perception of this concept to include a more holistic approach, one that includes balance and variety, you may avoid the pitfalls of volatile eating (also known as yo-yo dieting), and you may discover a more harmonious relationship with food and to yourself.

We seem to have an unparalleled obsession with health, yet North Americans are the most overweight, obese, and unhealthy people in the world. The polarity of health messages is intensifying—the more overweight our culture becomes, the more the media saturates us with images of "skinny." Worldwide, there are 1 billion people overweight and 1 billion people underweight; ironically, they are both malnourished. With the diet industry weighing in (pun intended) at an estimated $70 billion, its continued success proves that dieting is an ineffective way to lose weight, and, my guess is, only intensifies compulsive eating in most people. Studies show that 25 percent of American men and 45 percent of American women are on a diet on any given day.[18] More people are struggling with disordered eating than ever before. In the United States, as many as 10 million females and 1 million males are fighting a life-and-death battle with an eating disorder such as anorexia or bulimia, and approximately 25 million more are struggling with binge-eating disorder (or BED, characterized by a *"loss of control* over eating behaviors"), now the largest category of disordered eating, affecting up to 10 percent of the American population.[19] In addition, some 80 percent of American women are dissatisfied with their appearance.[20] There's even a new term used to describe an unhealthy obsession with being healthy—orthorexia—yet another disorder that is becoming more commonplace in our culture. This doesn't have to be the reality that we collectively create, and it certainly doesn't have to continue this way.

Obviously these diets don't work. What does the word "diet" actually mean? The word "diet" comes from the Latin word *diaeta,* meaning "a manner of living; a way of life." It was originally used to describe daily living, which includes what and how we eat. What and how we eat are a small part of the larger vision of an all-encompassing healthy lifestyle.

Even the very notion that you would have to embark on a radical regimen with the sole intention to lose weight is counter-productive. Through our dieting efforts, we've only become more removed from our natural way of being, but as I've discovered and will outline in this book, you can step off the dieting path altogether and end your struggle with food by reconnecting to your natural food source—Mother Earth—once again.

Misinformation Overload: Facing Away from Ourselves

Over time, as information has become highly specialized, we've shifted away from trusting our instincts and relied solely on information from external sources. Most of this information is tainted by the interests of people whose primary motivation is money and control—namely the food industry, the health industry, and the government, all of which have evolved into one big mess of contradictory information. Through aggressive marketing and advertising, these interests have convinced us that they are the only sources of valid nutritional information.

An overstimulating and stressful environment conditions us to scan this constant overload of information for answers and quick-fix solutions to our challenges in a vain search to "improve" ourselves as if we are incomplete, broken, and need fixing. As a result, we are constantly being bombarded with information aimed at influencing our behavior, which is the fundamental basis of advertising and marketing. But the marketing budget of big food companies promoting fake foods far outweighs the local organic farmers offering you the gift of real food. So in your search for answers, especially when you're desperate to try anything to end your struggle with food, you're more likely to be met with unsustainable, downright unhealthy solutions.

This constant search for answers to our food-related problems urges us to "turn away" from our inner intuitive guidance. What do I mean by "turn away?" It means that instead of being guided by our own inner knowing, we are searching outside of ourselves for the answer. We are sacrificing our health to achieve a culturally defined outer beauty and in the process are ruining our relationship with food, the very thing that can save us from this struggle. Magazine ads, television commercials, and billboards tell us that we *are not* okay, that we are broken, and that we need to do something—to buy something—to make us better. As a result, we often relate to our bodies on a superficial level, struggling to find something external to ourselves to make us happy, missing out on the wisdom that is already within us.

Getting Unhooked

We don't need more information, more numbers, more experts, or more ways to dissect the nutritional value of food. What we need is a more heartfelt *connection* to the invisible aspects of food that nourishes our entire being—not just our bodies. What we need is more meaning and more mindfulness surrounding what and how we eat. What we need is to change the way we *relate* to food and redefine what real food means to us, so that we can have a deeper connection to this miracle that is a part of our everyday lives. What's missing is a more conscious, intuitive way of relating to food, a reconnection to our inherent wisdom, our underlying intentions, and our food source.

Chapter 2

Unhooked: The Healing Process of Reconnection

In all honesty, our food environment makes it quite difficult for people to end their struggle with food. Recovering drug addicts never have to see or come into contact with their drug of choice again (if they successfully set up their environment in a supportive, drug-free way). But people who struggle with food—whether it's food addiction, a binge-eating disorder, compulsive overeating, food cravings, or an obsession with weight—simply do not have this same luxury of abstinence. We need to eat to survive. We can't cut out all the food from our lives and hope to stick around for much longer. Couple this with the confusion people feel about what they should eat to improve their health, combined with past failed attempts, I can understand how becoming "unhooked" from the struggle can feel slightly overwhelming.

We will get more food and nutrition specific in chapter 4, but for now, let's start with how you can set yourself up for success by making changes to and shifting your perception of your environment: both inner and outer. The good news is that the answers to health from a holistic and integrated lifestyle perspective are not as complicated as you might think. Many of the answers we seek regarding food and nutrition can be found in nature. This means looking past our fabricated, synthetic food environment, stripping away the layers of plastic packaging, and returning to our connection to the earth, leaving behind "diet mentality" once and for all. It's through this integrated reconnection process that true healing of our collective disordered and dysfunctional relationship with food can take place.

We align with this new paradigm when we radically shift the way we view and interact with our environment, operating from a place of *connectedness*, mending our previous disconnect. Reconnecting to our inner wisdom, to our underlying motivations, intentions, and perceptions, to a supportive social group, and most importantly, to our food source is the foundation upon which we can build better health.

Reconnecting to Your Inner Wisdom

A client came to me expressing discontent with her body. She, like many of my clients, had one primary goal: weight loss. She felt that she ate a healthy diet but was frustrated that she was still gaining weight. I asked her what a typical day of eating looked like—which is always a good place to start. She replied that she usually ate oats with milk for breakfast. I asked her how that food felt in her body, and after a long pause, she said that it made her feel tired, bloated, and gassy, and it didn't usually sit well in her stomach. I asked her why she ate that every morning, despite a clear message from her body not to consume that particular food. She paused for a second, and looked at me and said, "Because I was told oats were good for me."

This is a perfect example of something we all do: we allow our thinking mind to override our feeling body. Although it's important to gather information from trusted sources, we need to take our own inherent wisdom into account. We lived without nutritional experts telling us what to eat for hundreds of thousands of years; it's time we connect back to our instincts when it comes to what and how to eat.

What I'm proposing is an inside-out approach where you connect to your inherent wisdom and move outward from there, taking in information from the external environment but staying rooted within this inner awareness. Many of the practices in this book will help strengthen this connection to your *self*. Allow your dominant analytical mind to take a back seat, and give yourself permission to be guided by your heart and inner body wisdom.

Your body has an amazing ability to heal itself. Millions of different processes are currently taking place in your body that do not require your conscious thought for them to occur. Your heart automatically beats and your lungs expand and contract without you having to think about it; your hair and fingernails grow themselves; your immune system works wonders for you every single day. Your body is far more intelligent than your mind can ever grasp. When you recognize this, you can start to tap into the wealth of knowledge that your body possesses; root yourself in this knowing.

On your journey toward establishing a healthy relationship with food, you may need a guide, someone to help you along the way, but ultimately nobody can actually give you the answers you are looking for; you have all the answers you need. When seeking out information and help, always try to keep at least one foot in that pool of awareness. Start to pay attention, tune in, and listen to what your body is communicating to you. You are a walking, talking, living miracle, perfectly designed to know how much you should eat, sleep, and exercise. This is the best broadcast to tune into. Also start to notice the influence that magazines, television, billboard advertisements, the health food industry, your friends, and your family have on you, and remember to keep returning to your connection with your own truth.

Exercise: Is That My Food Craving or Inherent Wisdom Talking?

Having struggled with addiction to processed foods for many years, I know firsthand that it can be initially quite challenging to decipher between "inherent body wisdom" and an addiction-driven craving. If your body is screaming at you to *eat that cake!* how can you trust your inner wisdom? These are good questions to be asking. As I've come to realize, nature has our answers. A good place to start is by asking yourself a few simple questions to help you decipher whether this is a craving or your inner body awareness guiding you in the right direction:

1. Is this a real, whole food found in nature? Or is it a processed food product that is a result of food engineering?
2. Does eating this food make me feel out of control?
3. Am I genuinely hungry? Do I need this specific food, or could I eat another whole food instead?
4. Was my sudden appetite triggered by an internal or external cue that brought on a rapid shift from "not hungry" to "craving?"
5. Do feelings of guilt, shame, and blame follow after eating this food?

If your "inner body" is screaming for the usual food suspects—highly addictive foods that once you start eating them, it's hard for you to stop—then chances are this is a craving, not your inner body awareness guiding you to eat real food. Some may also be surprised to find out that cravings may be fueled by common food allergens, like wheat and soy, or an addiction to hyperpalatable foods high in sugar, fat, and salt. If you could easily reach for a banana or apple out of true genuine hunger instead of impulsively eating a food item that grabs your attention, then you're more likely to be genuinely hungry for food, not just trying to satisfy a craving. If you feel out of control, unable to stop, and feel down or depressed with feelings of guilt, shame, and blame after eating this food, that's another good sign this is your food-addicted brain screaming at you to get your fix.

Over time, it will get easier. I promise. Follow the guidelines in this book to become unhooked and free from the struggle, and you will slowly but surely allow yourself to tune into what your body actually wants, rather than what your cravings deceive you into believing you want.

Reconnect to Your Underlying Intentions:
Acting from a Place of Love

Long-lasting change is possible. To increase your chance of success, it's essential that you look at the underlying intentions that are motivating you. When your driving force is rooted in love (self-kindness, self-compassion, and self-love), as opposed to fear (self-criticism, self-denigration, and self-loathing), you build a solid foundation upon which to launch your success. True change is never possible when it is rooted in feelings of fear—fear of not being good enough, fear of not being loved, fear of failure. When you try to change from a place of "I'm not good enough exactly as I am," or "If I don't lose weight, nobody will love me," or "I will only be able to love myself when I'm at my desired weight," then positive long-lasting change will be more challenging. Trying to change for others creates a weak foundation. A strong, solid foundation for change is built on self-respect, self-care, and self-love.

In order to unhook yourself from the vise grip of addictive food, you need to find alternative ways to *feel good*, with many solutions offered throughout this book. You can feel completely differently doing the same action when you have two very different underlying intentions motivating that action. Take jogging, for example. If you go out and jog with a positive intention rooted in self-love and self-care, and it comes from a place of "I'm motivated to strengthen my body because I have so much love and respect for the miracle of my body and want to express that miracle through movement," you will feel better than if it comes from a place of "I'm overweight, I don't really like to jog—actually, I hate jogging, but I know I should do it because I need to lose weight, because I'm not good enough as I am." Can you see the difference? The second scenario requires struggling to push through, but the first one doesn't; it's just a natural extension of loving your body and wanting to move it because it makes you happy.

I'll never forget the day that I had this completely clear insight—that everything I did was rooted in this fearful existence of not being good enough. That's why establishing lasting change was difficult for me for so many years—my motivation didn't have a solid foundation. I had to reevaluate everything in my life and ask myself why I was doing it, for whom I was doing it, and whether it was rooted in love or fear. This allowed me to come back to doing things that felt good and that I enjoyed.

Reconnect to Your Underlying Motivations

At what point in your life did you hit your rock-bottom moment? What did that moment look like or, more importantly, *feel* like for you? It might have been the time you stepped on the scale and it pushed past two hundred pounds, or the moment your son's best friend called you a cow, or the time you locked yourself in the bathroom to binge in private and you caught a glimpse of yourself in the mirror. It could be a flash moment of awareness that you're totally obsessed and consumed with thoughts of food and of all the pain and suffering it's causing you.

You might be familiar with rock bottom: that place where the pain of staying the same and hooked (depressed, unhappy, obsessed with food, struggling with overeating, counting calories, etc.) now outweighs the pain of change and becoming unhooked (changing your lifestyle, withdrawal from addictive foods, losing the weight, exercising, etc. . . .) Rock bottom is a painful place to be; however, it can also become, if used wisely, a strong impetus for change. It's the point where you absolutely know that you can no longer go on living this way. And the best part about hitting rock bottom? The only place you have to go from there is up.

I had countless moments of embarrassment—yes we can have multiple rock-bottom moments—like the time I was walking down the hallway in high school, and a boy shouted out to everyone that my butt was getting bigger by the day. Or the many times I decided to stay home instead of going out and socializing because I felt horrible in my own body. Or the time I binged and purged so many times in a day that my faced swelled up to the point where I hardly recognized myself. These were all difficult and painful moments to endure, but I remember one moment in particular that really hit it home for me.

When I was in group therapy for women with eating disorders, I met an older woman I will call Katie. She was about fifty years old at the time, and it was very apparent that her cognitive function was very poor, based on her inability to focus or complete a sentence properly. She told us she had been starving herself for over thirty years and what hell it had been for her. It was in that moment that it hit me: I realized that if I kept putting off making changes until tomorrow or next week, I would end up like her—fifty years into my life and still struggling with food and weight issues. As a result, Katie became one of my motivations for change. I then wrote her name on several cards and placed them in various strategic places to remind me of my motivation. I also made a list of all my other positive motivators, like being more social, feeling comfortable in my body, and fitting into some of my favorite clothes again, and added new motivators to the list on a regular basis.

Exercise: Identifying Your Motivation

Get out your journal or a piece of paper and a pen and answer the following questions. Don't overthink the questions; simply write whatever comes to you:

1. What was your rock-bottom moment? Briefly describe when you realized that continuing to make unhealthy choices did not align with your deeper desire of living a healthy, balanced lifestyle. Which moment sticks out for you in particular?
2. Make a list of all the emotions you were feeling at that point in your life.
3. Now make a list of all the things you want to feel as a result of being free of this struggle.
4. What are your motivations for change?
5. How can you remind yourself of these motivators?

Reconnect to Nature

For those of you who know what it's like to struggle with food—or who struggle with any addiction, for that matter—you know how much time can be spent focusing on "the problem." It's like we get caught in a loop, and around and around we go. One very effective way that you can make your environment work for you rather than against you and help break that downward spiraling cycle is to go outside and spend time in nature. Nature has a calming effect on us and can help improve memory and attention span, according to new research from the University of Michigan.[21] According to one of the researchers, Marc Berman, "interacting with nature can have similar effects as meditating." Favor time in nature over time with technology to help reduce stress and make you feel good in your body and your mind.

We are meant to spend time outside and be exposed to mood-enhancing vitamin D from the sun, fresh air and oxygen from the trees, and the visual pleasures of different natural landscapes. Now, most people live in an environment not only predominated by synthetic food, but also by artificial lighting and electronics, and are inundated with electromagnetic frequencies. This plays a role in disorienting our natural circadian rhythms and influencing our "time awareness," as noted in the report "Healthy Parks, Healthy People," issued by the Deakin University School of Health and Social Development in Melbourne, Australia:[22]

> City life is dominated by mechanical time (punctuality, deadlines, etc.), yet our bodies and minds are dominated by biological time. Conflicts between mechanical and biological time can result in a variety of unpleasant psychosomatic symptoms, including irritability, restlessness, depression, insomnia, tension and headaches, and indigestion (Furnass, 1979). If unaddressed, these problems have the potential to eventuate into illnesses that are more serious. The experience of nature in a neurological sense can help strengthen the activities of the right hemisphere of the brain, and restore harmony to the functions of the brain as a whole (Furnass, 1979). This is perhaps a technical explanation of the process that occurs when people "clear their head" by going for a walk in a park . . .

Make an effort to open the windows in your house, get outside for a walk, and eat fresh, water-rich food in its whole, natural, organic state. Turn off your computer and electronic devices in the evening and allow time to adjust and align with the natural rhythms of the sun and moon.

You may be surprised to hear that physically connecting to the earth and, specifically, walking barefoot on the earth (a rapidly growing field of study called "earthing" or "grounding") can have major health benefits. According to Stephen

Sinatra, MD, a co-author of *Earthing: The Most Important Health Discovery Ever?*, "The earth's surface is negatively charged and has an unlimited supply of 'free electrons.' If your body has lots of positively charged free radicals (creating inflammation), the earth's free electrons can help to neutralize them. When our feet or our bodies touch the ground, electrons naturally flow from the place where they are plentiful (the earth) to where they are not (our bodies)."[23] According to Dr. James Oschman, PhD, an expert in the field of energy medicine, these free electrons are probably the most potent antioxidants known to man. This connection results specifically in beneficial changes in heart rate, decreased levels of inflammation, a boost to the immune system, reduction in stress hormones, and returning the human body to its most natural electrical state.[24]

Most people live in cities surrounded by pavement and cover their feet with shoes, and therefore rarely make physical contact with the earth. This was not how our bodies were designed to live, and the effect of living in this modern world is taking its toll. In order to enjoy the benefits of reconnecting with nature, take time at least once a day to make contact! Get your feet dirty; walk around on the grass in your yard, in a park, or on the sand at the beach. Make an effort—it will do your body, mind, and spirit a world of good.

Perhaps the use of the word "reconnect" is not the best choice of words here because it implies that we are "disconnected." Although in one way, we are extremely far removed from nature, we are not literally disconnected, that would be impossible. We are not separate from nature—we *are* nature. We are but a thread woven into the fabric we call nature—it is the fiber that holds all our souls together. So it's not so much about reconnecting as it is about re-attuning to and remembering our inherent oneness with the earth and eating and living in a way that reflects that. Reconnecting in the sense of remembering means to "know something again" as if for the first time.

"The earth has music for those who listen."

—William Shakespeare

Reconnect to Your Food Source

When giving interviews or conducting workshops I am often asked: "What is the most powerful way to mend our relationship with food?" From my perspective, two of the most important factors are connecting with our food source and incorporating mindfulness and meditation into our lives (which I discuss in chapter 10).

One of the most significant events that helped me heal my disordered relationship with food was learning how to grow my food. Gardening helped save my life. Watching food grow and taking part in the process is nothing short of awe inspiring. As I touched the vine that grew the tomatoes I loved so much, picked cherries and ate them right off the tree, and fell in love with my cucumber plants, I developed a direct connection with life—*my life*. I came to realize that the food I was eating, right from the ground, was providing me with the energy I needed to sustain my life, to wake up in the morning and go for a walk, and to do the things I loved to do. This triggered a series of self-inquiring questions. What am I doing with this energy? Am I truly appreciating this gift of sustenance? Am I doing something of importance to benefit the greater good? Or am I going to continue wallowing in my own self-absorbed struggle? I gained a whole new appreciation for the precious moments in my life that I had previously failed to acknowledge and even took for granted.

We learn to respect all living matter and recognize the earth as a living, breathing organism through the reconnection process. Once we recognize and remember this connection we share with nature and our food source, so many other areas of our lives naturally shift to support a healthier way of living and *being*. When we develop a relationship with where our food comes from, we start to shift our relationship not only to food but also to ourselves and to our bodies. This is where healing our relationship with food begins: literally from the ground up.

Everyone has the capacity to reconnect to their food source on some level. No need to quit your job and dedicate your life to "living off the land" to enjoy the simple pleasures of reconnecting to where your food comes from. Growing a garden is wonderful, and I recognize not everyone has the time (or desire) to do this. There are many options for those who do, like renting a small garden plot in a community garden (urban gardening is now thriving in many cities across North America), starting a potted garden on your balcony or an herb garden on your windowsill, or simply growing sprouts in your kitchen. You may want to explore visiting a local farm—or better yet, volunteering on an organic farm (check out Willing Workers on Organic Farms for great opportunities to travel and learn how to grow your own food).

Do not underestimate the power of this reconnection with real, whole food. We have an internship program that we run here in Hawaii that teaches how to live in harmony with the earth, grow food, and create delicious meals, coupled with mindful eating and nutritional education. Nature is our ultimate healer. I'm reminded of this when I see one of our program interns crying in the garden. These are tears of remembering what many have long forgotten about their inherent connection to nature and, perhaps more importantly, about their self worth; they are tears of coming home to oneself.

Reconnect to a Healthy Environment: Minimizing Triggers

Everywhere we look there are billboards and commercials portraying packaged, processed foods, and there are fast-food restaurants and convenience stores on every corner. These visual cues trigger us to crave and desire foods even when we're not hungry. If we are constantly triggered to eat because of cues in our environment, can we rework our environment to cue us to eat more healthfully and less of the foods that keep us hooked? Although it would be difficult to tear down every last billboard with images of burgers and fries or simply walk around with blinders on, we can indeed make small changes in our immediate environment that add up to big results. Let's start off in the kitchen.

Making Friends with Your Kitchen

According to the Bureau of Labor Statistics, in 2012 the average person spent about 40 percent of their food dollars in restaurants. Restaurants are the perfect food-trigger environment, with large and sometimes unlimited portions, and foods loaded with sugar, fat, and salt that make it difficult to stop eating despite how full we are. When was the last time you left a restaurant feeling only comfortably full and not overstuffed? Remember that restaurants are in the business of making repeat customers out of us. We also don't have control over the quality of ingredients that they use, or know what ingredients they use, for that matter.

Transitioning to a healthy lifestyle requires that you make friends with your kitchen and learn how to make delicious and nutritious meals. Eating healthy is easier and not as time consuming as you may think, but it does require a little time and energy to learn how to feed yourself properly (more on this in chapter 4).

The setup of your kitchen will impact what you choose to eat and how much. Let's look at some simple ways you can set up your kitchen environment to cue you to eat less and eat healthier:

- **Downsize the dishware.** First off, take a look at your dishware. The average dinner plate is 11 to 12 inches wide, a drastic increase from the standard 8- to 9-inch plate from only a few decades ago. If you're consistently overeating and are a part of the "clean your plate" club, then consider downsizing your dishware. Using a bigger plate can add another 250 calories to an "average" standard American meal every day; that's an extra 26 pounds per year! You can keep your larger plates for your fruit- and vegetable-based meals to encourage you to eat more of these low-calorie, nutrient-dense foods.

- **Drink out of tall narrow glasses.** Most people tend to underestimate how many calories they consume from beverages. What kind of beverages do you drink? I recommend drinking as much water, coconut water, fresh green juices, and herbal teas as you care for and keep other drinks like refined fruit juices and sodas to a bare minimum. Better yet, consider phasing them out completely. Visually, we tend to measure things by height, not width, so it's easy to underestimate how much we pour into short, wide glasses compared to tall, narrow glasses. If you are going to continue to drink store-bought beverages, at least replace your short, wide glasses for tall, narrow glasses to encourage yourself to consume less processed drinks with refined sugar and caffeine.

- **Make your most useful kitchen tools easily accessible.** I use my blender multiple times a day, as whole food smoothies, fresh raw soups, homemade salad dressings, dips, and delicious sauces have become a mainstay in my dietary lifestyle. The same goes for my juicer, as I love to make fresh vegetable juices. I dedicate prime counter space to permanently park these health-supporting kitchen essentials to encourage easy access, as I use them frequently. Consider what is occupying your counter space and get the tools you need (a high-powered blender and juicer is a good place to start) to help support you on your journey to health. Do you really need your microwave occupying prime counter space? What about your coffee machine? Scan your countertops and see what you can replace with more health-supporting kitchen tools.

- **Remove trigger foods.** Every time we see food that we crave, we are triggered to eat it. Make a list of all the foods that you find difficult to stop eating once you start. These are the foods that torment you, the ones that make you feel out of control or feel guilty after you eat them. These are usually processed foods high in sugar, fat, and salt: chips, cookies, donuts, chocolate, or ice cream. For some it could be bread or pasta, processed peanut butter, or Twinkies. Get a garbage bag and remove all the fake foods from your house. Don't feel bad; feel empowered—better in the garbage than in your body! Once out of sight, it's easier to keep out of mind.

- **Remove processed food.** Look at the food in your fridge and in your cupboards. Look at the bottles, jars, and packages of foods, especially ones that have been there for a very long time. Why is it they haven't gone bad yet? What preservatives are in these products that are preventing the natural lifecycle of foods to take place? Do you really want to be consuming these unnatural "shelf life" foods? Check out their labels; do you recognize the ingredients? If not, consider removing it from your kitchen—and your diet.

- **Buy in bulk—fruits and veggies only.** Start stocking your fridge with lots of organic fruits and vegetables, locally grown if possible. These are the foods you want to focus on buying in bulk (although, you might prefer making more frequent trips to the store to avoid food spoilage), and skip the enormous multipack fake foods to prevent overeating.

- **Repackage into small serving sizes.** If you're not quite willing to part with some of your favorite snack foods and you do choose to buy snack foods that come in bigger packages, downsize them into smaller portion sizes, preventing you from overeating or eating the whole package in one sitting.

- **Make healthy food the most convenient.** We naturally want things to be as easy and effortless as possible, so make eating healthy easy! Fruit and vegetables have to be the original definition of "fast food." What's easier than peeling a banana or washing an apple and eating it? Place a big bowl of fruit on your counter of your kitchen table. Place your fruits and vegetables in plain sight in the front of your fridge, and less healthy foods (if you must have them there) in the back.

Here are a few other quick tips to prevent you from overeating while either snacking alone or eating meals with others:

- **Minimize distractions.** When you eat, simply eat without combining it with other activities like watching TV or reading. Just enjoy the food you have in front of you. If you are eating with other people and are feeling distracted, keep coming back to your awareness of eating.

- **Minimize variety.** When you're at a social event or having people over, remember the studies about variety: the more variety, the more likely you are to overeat. Our bodies were designed to eat very simply, only one or two foods at a sitting—and I don't mean one or two dishes with fifteen ingredients each! I mean one or two whole foods. Start to notice if you load up more because of variety, and consciously choose to put a minimal number of foods on your plate at a time.

- **Get the food off the table**. When you're serving dinner, don't leave food on the table; leave it in the kitchen where it's out of immediate reach. This simple act will increase the effort a person needs to make to get the food and is more likely to reduce consumption.

- **Avoid eating from the package**. If you're about to eat a snack from the package, put the portion you plan to eat on a plate and put the rest of the package away.

- **Ask yourself: Am I really hungry?** Because eating with others influences our eating decisions, halfway through your meal, ask yourself: "Am I still hungry, or am I just eating because everyone else is?"

- **Point in the right direction, then go at your own pace.** Some people like to jump right in to making changes; others prefer to take smaller steps. If you eat out five times a week, aim to eat out one or two times per week. If it feels good for you, try eating out only once a month, and if you're willing to jump right in, save restaurants for rare and special occasions only. If you eat one portion of fruit per day, try to increase that to two or three. Try incorporating a fruit smoothie a couple of mornings per week, and work your way up from there. By increasing the fresh foods in your healthy lifestyle, you'll likely have less room for and less desire for the packaged, processed foods.

Reconnect to New Perceptions

Our inner thoughts and perceptions change the way we look at the world. When I was learning to unhook myself from an unhealthy lifestyle, I did not expect the government to step in and start regulating our out-of-control food environment or start tearing down fast-food restaurants by the dozen. I needed to use the power of my own mind and consciously shift my perceptions to help unhook me from what were once my cravings. As I transitioned to a healthy lifestyle, my perceptions of these foods naturally changed over time, but you can also prompt a shift in perspective to initiate the changes that you want to make.

Where I once used to crave and desire the foods that kept me hooked, I now look at those foods with utter disgust; thinking about eating those greasy, (literally) sickening foods makes me feel queasy in my stomach. The more I learn about what's actually in new food products, the more I view them as science experiments—and we're the guinea pigs! At the same time, I started looking at whole foods and noticing how beautiful and colorful they looked and how delicious and juicy they tasted. It was a process of re-scripting my thought process, perceptions, and belief systems about the food I was eating. This is how we can use the power of perception to unhook ourselves from craving and internal struggle and connect to freedom from desire.

Reconnect to a Positive and Supportive Social Network

I'll never forget the first time I watched Dan Buettner's Ted.com talk on "How to Live to Be 100+." So many people are searching for the secrets to longevity, yet are focused predominantly on nutrition. "Do the longest-lived people eat a lot of omega-3s in fish? Do they eat dairy? Do they follow high-fat or low-fat diets? What about yogurt, is that the key? Do they consume meat or only fish?"

But as it turns out, and as Dan Buettner describes, there isn't one singular dietary formula, although there are general dietary patterns seen in these areas that Buettner calls "blue zones." He coined the term to refer to the areas where people tend to live longer, healthier lives with fewer diseases. All the "blue zones" had nine traits in common with only a couple of them actually related to food: a diet lighter on meat and excess calories and heavier on plants, daily physical activity, effective stress management, rare overeating, a strong sense of purpose, participating in some kind of spiritual or faith-based practice, and a strong social support network of friends and families. The non-food related factors, like having a strong social network, are just as important as what one chooses to eat. All of these cultures also cultivated a strong connection to the earth and experienced low levels of depression.

As the research from the "blue zones" shows, it is important to have a strong social support group, and to surround yourself with people who have a positive influence on you. Research from the ongoing Framingham Studies started in 1948 shows that smoking, obesity, happiness, and even loneliness are contagious. The people you socialize with can have a big impact on your health and can also influence how much you weigh. One study published in the *New England Journal of Medicine*[25] involved a detailed analysis of a large social network of 12,067 people who were closely followed for 32 years (from 1971 until 2003). The researchers recorded the weight of the participants at various times over the course of the study, as well as the weights of their friends, spouses, siblings, and neighbors. The results are striking:

- Chances of becoming obese increase by about 57 percent when a friend became obese.
- Friends had more of an influence than family members on weight.
- Influence of friends remained despite large geographic distance.
- The greatest influence of all was between mutual close friends. There, if one became obese, the other had a 171 percent increased chance of becoming obese too.
- If one spouse became obese, the likelihood that the other spouse would become obese increased by 37 percent.
- Persons of the same sex had relatively greater influence on each other than those of the opposite sex.
- Neighbors had no influence.

Are you surprised by the power of your social connections? Our friends influence our perceptions and what we consider as appropriate behavior. That's why if you're dining with people who overeat, you're likely to overeat as well. If everyone around you becomes obese, it is viewed as more socially acceptable. According to Dr. Nicholas Christakis, a physician and professor of medical sociology at Harvard Medical School and a principal investigator in the study: "You change your idea of what is an acceptable body type by looking at the people around you."

The good news is that the same occurs for weight loss, although it's less predominant because in our culture, more people tend to be gaining weight than losing weight. The same applies to happiness. If you have a friend living within a mile of you, and that friend becomes happy, you have a 25 percent greater probability of becoming happy yourself.[26] This doesn't mean you should ditch your unhealthy, unhappy friends; we are social beings by nature, and friends are also an important part of our sense of well-being. But we shouldn't underestimate the influence that our friends and family have on us. Social isolation is linked to depression,[27] and even heart disease.[28]

Here are a few tips to help you with your social support group:

- **Know who your negative enablers are.** These are the people you spend time with who enable you to eat more than you otherwise would, or influence you to make unhealthy choices. They influence you to skip the gym and watch a movie instead, take the escalator instead of the stairs, and order the double cheeseburger instead of a salad. Start to notice who these people are and how much time you spend with them. Sometimes our enablers can be close to home, or in our home. This doesn't mean that you need to get a divorce or give up your kids for adoption; just start to notice how much you're influenced by those around you and pay special attention to who can influence you towards a healthier lifestyle. Remember that you can be the seed of change in your social network and household, acting as a *positive* enabler for your friends and family.

- **Surround yourself with people who are healthy.** When you start living a healthier lifestyle, you're naturally going to gravitate towards people who encourage you to be healthy. Making friends and hanging out with people with similar health goals can help support, encourage, and influence you to improve your health. Consider taking up a yoga class or joining a gym to make new social contacts, or perhaps speaking with a health coach.

- **Connect with like-minded people.** One of the reasons that twelve-step programs work so well is because they connect with, offer, and receive support from other people who understand what they're going through. If you are struggling with disordered eating, even if it's not a medically defined eating disorder, reach out and connect with others who are also in recovery and healing mode. It's important that they are firmly rooted on the path of recovery so they do not become negative enablers. There are organizations like Food Addicts Anonymous and Overeaters Anonymous, as well as many others that help people with specific issues like binge eating, bulimia, anorexia, or being overweight or obese.

- **Enroll your family.** One of the most frequent complaints among my female clients is that they are trying to make changes at home, but their families are still making unhealthy choices, making it more difficult to follow through on change. Get the support of your partner and/or children and ask for their help. Tell them you're making changes and would like their moral support. Make this a journey that you can embark on together. Take healthy cooking classes together, learn to make new recipes together, or enroll in an online course geared towards healthy living and go through the course as a family. Take your family on a health adventure vacation, where you can have fun and immerse yourself in learning healthy lifestyle skills to bring home with you. There are wonderful health-focused family vacations all over the world, including our raw food Hawaii vacations and retreats. (Check out www. happyandraw.com for our upcoming events.)

- **Join healthy social media networks.** Considering how many hours a day the average person spends on social media networks like Twitter, Facebook, and Pinterest, it's worth putting that time to good use to help fuel your healthy lifestyle! Connect with people via social media to share healthy recipes, exercise tips, and daily bits of motivational inspiration. Better yet, you can skip the computer and join in face-to-face social groups through organizations like MeetUp.com to locate other individuals in your area that share a similar interest in healthy living. There are groups created in major cities all over the world for vegans, vegetarians, and raw foodies, and also for people who share activity interests like hiking, walking, running, swimming, biking, dancing, etc.

Off the Hook

Positive change starts to happen when you actively create an environment that is supportive of the changes you want to make. Through this process it's important to stay connected to your inner wisdom and really look at your underlying intentions and motivations, as well as question your beliefs and perceptions around "healthy" and "unhealthy" food. Reconnecting to your natural food source in some way can offer you profound insights and help you shift these perceptions to be more supportive of a healthy lifestyle. Spending more time in nature, making more meals at home, and surrounding yourself with a positive social network are all ways that you can set up a strong foundation for change. This is the beginning of laying a new path to freedom from the struggle.

For me, being caught in the food struggle was like being imprisoned in a small dark room—and I didn't think I was ever going to get out. But as I started researching and understanding what was going on in my body when I was eating these highly addictive foods, I was astonished. I was able to take one big sigh of relief because I realized I was not a complete moral failure with zero willpower. I was hooked and didn't even know it—and many others don't know it either. In Part Two, we will cover the concept of food addiction from a physiological perspective and explore what's really taking place in our bodies when we eat processed foods—the staple of the American diet.

PART TWO

The Physiological Hook

"But where the links between eating and drugs get really interesting is in the brain. There, narcotics and food—especially food that is high in salt, sugar, and fat—act much alike. Once ingested, they race along the same pathways, using the same neurological circuitry to reach the brain's pleasure zones, those areas that reward us with enjoyable feelings for doing the right thing by our bodies. Or, as the case may be, for doing what the brain has been led to believe is the right thing."
—**Michael Moss,** *Salt Sugar Fat: How the Food Giants Hooked Us*

Chapter 3

How Our Physiology Hooks Us

Our food environment has changed in terms of how much food is available, where it's available, and when it's available, but most importantly, it's changed in terms of *what* is available. As we discussed in chapter 1, processed foods predominate in our current environment. Most of what is available to us has been refined down to the point that it now more closely resembles a drug than a nutrient-dense, real food. These "hyper-palatable" foods, a term used in the food industry to refer to foods abnormally high in sugar, fat, and salt,* are literally taking over the natural processes of the brain and are contributing to the development of chronic overeating and food addiction.

The Big Three: Sugar, Fat, and Salt

Take a moment to think about the foods you crave. What do they all have in common? What is it about these foods that trigger you to eat them when you're not

---

* Although the use of the term "hyper-palatable" food is used by the food industry, perhaps a more appropriate term would be "hyper-stimulating." I personally think of fruit as *highly* palatable; there's nothing more palatable to me than my favorite fresh, ripe fruit. Keep in mind that "hyper-palatable" isn't used to describe whole foods; it's used by the food companies themselves to describe the hyper-stimulating effects that processed foods high in sugar, fat, and salt have on the brain. I will continue to use the term "hyper-palatable" as defined by the food industry.

41

hungry and to continue consuming them past fullness? Food addiction is generally related to refined, processed foods. Why is that? Besides the fact that these foods are replete with chemicals, food additives, preservatives, and neurotoxins—oh, and don't forget genetic modification—these processed foods have three very important ingredients in common: refined *sugar, fat, and salt*.

You may be thinking that these are three natural ingredients that have been used in food preparation for many years. Sugar, fat, and salt are not inherently the problem, at least not in the combinations found in nature. It turns out that the food industry is combining these three ingredients in extreme ratios that are *not normally* found in nature, and this results in a mismatch between our food environment and our biology. What is it about sugar, fat, and salt that has changed? Quality and quantity. With the advent of food engineering, the result of altering the quality and quantity of sugar, fat, and salt in the majority of the twenty thousand new food products that hit the shelves each year has led the average American to consume a diet predominated by refined foods, especially refined carbohydrates, fats, and salt.

1. **Quality.** Due to the for-profit nature of the food industry, there is a continual search to reduce product costs and source out cheaper ingredients. This in turn drives the quality of food ingredients down. Due to food technology and the refining process, the quality of these foods have drastically declined. As we will discuss, our bodies process and digest refined substances very differently than food in its whole state.

2. **Quantity.** This is a twofold problem. The quantity of these foods that we have access to and that make up our food environment is unprecedented. We are not biologically designed to live in an environment where food is available 24/7. We are biologically hardwired to seek out and consume sugar, fat, and salt as they are essential to our survival, but historically, there were famines and times of the year where these nutrients were relatively scarce.

Secondly, the sheer *amount* of the sugar, fat, and salt being *combined* into one food is literally taking over normal brain functioning. It's not just the sugar alone or the fat or salt alone that makes people want to keep eating, but a specific combination of them that really does the trick. Food companies have invested billions of dollars into finding the perfect "bliss point"—the exact amount of sweetness that will provide us with the maximum pleasure,[29] coupled with the perfect combination of fat, and salt, influencing our eating choices—much more than we realize.

Why We Overeat: The Balance of Two Systems

There are literally millions of processes going on in your body at any given time. Within this dynamic and ever-changing internal environment, your intelligent body is always striving to find homeostasis (a term for *balance*) to create a stable environment for your cells to grow and thrive. The regulation of body temperature and blood sugar levels are two examples of processes in the body that self-regulate to maintain balance, constantly adjusting to new information from other physiological processes.

Energy Balance and Homeostasis

Energy balance is another physiological process in your body regulated by homeostasis. This system guides your body to know when to eat and, more importantly, when to stop eating. When your energy stores are getting low, it sends a signal to your brain—the part of the brain that regulates energy balance—and then physical symptoms manifest to let you know it's time to eat and *motivates* you to seek out food. When you respond to these signals by eating, other signals are sent to your brain that tells you that you've had enough. Sounds simple, doesn't it? Wouldn't it be nice to be regulated in such an easy fashion? After all, our bodies are designed to be regulated by our inherent body wisdom of energy balance. And when our dietary lifestyle consists of real, whole foods—generally, we are.

Hedonic (Pleasure) Reward System

What would life be without a little pleasure? To complement the regulation of energy balance, we also have a hedonic or pleasure system made up of a collection of brain structures that influences behavior by inducing pleasurable effects and reinforces behaviors that prove to be "pleasurable." This just so happens to influence what we eat, how much we eat, when we start eating, and when we stop eating. Thankfully pleasure was granted to us as a very important survival mechanism to *reinforce* that we should repeat certain behaviors that feel good. This is part of the reason we are driven to eat. When we eat and engage in other important acts of survival like sex or social contact, our brain releases neurochemicals that are linked to the *reward system*, encouraging us to seek out these pleasurable acts, as a built-in mechanism to ensure the survival of the species.

Research shows that the reward-based regulation system can override the homeostatic process during periods of relative abundance by increasing the desire to consume foods that are hyper-palatable.[30] And which foods are the most hyper-palatable? You guessed it: processed foods that are exorbitantly high in sugar, fat, and salt. And guess what—they're everywhere. In other words, because these high-sugar, high-fat, high-salt foods *excite* and *stimulate* the pleasure center in our brain, they are effectively overriding the natural regulatory balance that is maintained when consuming real whole foods. As a consequence, this hedonic (pleasure) driven food intake is often reinforced; eating hyper-palatable foods for pleasure makes consumption even more likely in the future[31] and habitual behavioral patterns are reinforced.

A Taste for Addiction

I've worked with many overweight clients who would like nothing more than to drop their excess weight, but they say they are addicted to the *taste* of food. Can these addictive behaviors and chronic overeating be a result of the taste of food? Taste happens to evoke a stronger physiological and emotional response than the other senses. Interestingly enough, our taste buds have a direct line of communication to the pleasure center in the brain—and the food industry knows it. Eating food combinations disproportionately high in sugar, fat, and salt (and many other chemical ingredients) results in the stimulation of a wider range of neurons in each bite than simply biting into an apple. Basically these *hyper*-palatable foods are producing a *hyper*-pleasurable response in the brain's pleasure centers, which is very different than the way the brain responds when we eat simple, whole foods.

"[Food products] are knowingly designed—engineered is the better word—to maximize their allure. The packaging is tailored to excite our kids. Their advertising uses every psychological trick to overcome any logical arguments we might have for passing the product by. Their taste is so powerful, we remember it from the last time we walked down the aisle and succumbed, snatching them up. And above all else, their formulas are calculated and perfected by scientists who know very well what they are doing. The most crucial point to know is that there is nothing accidental in the grocery store. All of this is done with a purpose."

—**Michael Moss**, *Salt Sugar Fat*

When the brain's pleasure center is viewed through an fMRI while someone is eating these "rewarding" hyper-palatable foods, neurons show a preference for these particular foods because the brain's pleasure center lights up like a Christmas tree, similar to the brain of someone who is addicted to drugs. This is because the neural circuits implicated in drug conditioning, craving, and relapse overlap extensively with those involved in natural reward and reinforcement like food.[32] Some research even suggests that the intense sweetness of refined sugar surpasses the intense and strongly addictive high of cocaine reward.[33] If we see something that we want (whether it's ice cream or cocaine) and our brain lights up in response, the more likely we are going to crave and want to pursue the object of our desire.

The Feel-Good Chemicals

We are naturally driven by reward: the reward of pleasure. When you take part in pleasant activities, like connecting with loved ones, laughing with friends, eating a mango, walking in the park, or watching the sunrise over the ocean, your brain releases feel-good chemicals, giving you that warm and fuzzy feeling inside. These feelings of contentment, happiness, and peacefulness are what we all want to feel and naturally strive for.

The feel-good chemicals that trigger the pleasure response are dopamine and *opioids* (sound familiar?). Opioids are a category of brain chemicals, also known as endorphins, which produce similar effects to opiate drugs such as morphine and heroin. Endorphins give relief from pain, make us feel good, and give us a sensation of pleasure—it's our naturally produced morphine. Dopamine is another neurotransmitter that plays a number of roles associated to pleasurable reward, triggering feelings of satisfaction, happiness, and pleasure, and as we will also discuss, it influences what we focus our attention on. The dopamine and opioid systems are largely interconnected and play a significant role in our eating patterns.

We live in a culture where we are increasingly habituated to *over*stimulation (through food, television, advertising, loud music, etc.), and all this stimulation is amplifying the pleasurable response in the brain. The first time someone consumes high-sugar, high-fat, high-salt foods, they get an opioid and dopamine rush unlike anything they've ever felt in the past, closely resembling the pattern of opioid release seen in the brains of drug users.[34]

Opioids are not the only endorphins weighing into the mix. Other endorphins stimulate us to keep eating and are responsible for developing food cravings. Refined sugar and starch intake stimulates endorphin secretion. Beta-endorphin is produced by the pituitary gland and is reported to produce a more intense sense of well-being than any of the other endorphin types.[35] When we eat refined sugar, beta-endorphin is released, triggering the urge to eat more sugar, creating a snowball effect.[36] Dynorphin, another endorphin and powerful appetite stimulant, also increases the craving to eat, especially during stressful situations.[37]

All these feel-good chemicals have associated receptor sites in the brain that they can lock into; this is how the message of pleasure is relayed to the brain. Nora Volkow, MD, a pioneer in the study of food addiction and director of the National Institute of Drug Abuse (NIDA), has found that obese people have far fewer dopamine receptor sites in the brain's reward center, similar to the changes seen in the brain of drug addicts, and suggests that it's this decrease in the number of receptor sites that influences the development of food addiction. When your brain is constantly being inundated with tidal waves of pleasure chemicals, in its effort to try to maintain balance, the brain compensates by decreasing the number of dopamine receptor sites. This creates an interesting predicament: the fewer receptor sites, the more you need to consume to get that initial "high" from your first "fix." Additionally, it also becomes increasingly difficult to experience pleasure from the "simple" things in life, and a dull numbing can occur to life's greatest natural gifts, like seeing a baby smile or a flower blossoming. The good news is that our brain is highly adaptive to change, and with focused effort these receptor sites can be rebuilt over time. This requires unhooking yourself from the grip of hyper-palatable food, returning to a whole foods lifestyle, and incorporating the many recommendations throughout this book to boost your feel-good chemicals naturally.

Pause & Reflect: Exploring Your Relationship with Food

Take a moment to pause and turn your attention inward. Take a deep breath in, and slowly let it out with a big sigh, letting go and releasing any tension you may be holding onto in your body. Allow yourself the time and opportunity to reflect on the following questions:

1. Do I often want to stop eating but find it difficult to stop?
2. Am I often preoccupied with thoughts of food and weight?
3. Do I sometimes hide what I eat from other people or eat in secrecy?

4. Do I experience emotions such as guilt, shame, or sadness when I think about my relationship with food? Do I experience these feelings after I've eaten?
5. Do I fluctuate widely between binging and restricting?
6. Do I often eat past the point of comfortable fullness?
7. Have I tried to give up certain foods but cannot?
8. Do I continue to consume certain foods despite physical or emotional problems related to eating?

The Motivation to Eat

Up to this point we've discussed the pleasure system in the brain as a result of *eating* food, so why is it that *before* we've even put that food in our mouth we want or crave it, and become very motivated to satisfy that desire? I know I've gone to great lengths to fulfill a food craving, and even greater lengths to cover my tracks. Maybe you've hidden a chocolate bar wrapper or two in your day—but there's no need to hide away in shameful secrecy anymore. What we are doing in these pages is exposing the truth of the hidden lure of these foods.

There are very powerful biological factors at play that make us *want* a certain food enough to pursue it and then make us feel *momentarily* better once we obtain it.[38] This motivation and pursuit of food is a different set of processes taking place in our brain and body than the actual pleasure we gain from eating food, but they are interconnected.

Imagine you are walking through a beautiful forest. You are all alone and hungry. You see a branch overhead loaded with blackberries. Something inside you kicks into gear and drives you—*motivates you*—to seek out this food, the most primal of instinctual urges. If you've ever been really hungry and felt the effects of low blood sugar, you may know what I'm talking about. It's as if a separate entity inhabits your body, overpowers your rational mind, and overwhelms you with the ravenous desire to eat. Your body's instincts have taken over. What is it that's motivating this desire?

Through experience we learn to anticipate a reward, and it is this *anticipation* that provides motivation to act. Not only is dopamine responsible for pleasure felt, but it is also responsible for grabbing our attention and helping us to focus on something—*but on what?*

If I show you a picture of a piece of chocolate cake next to a picture of celery sticks, you're likely to gravitate toward the chocolate cake. Chocolate will grab your attention more than the celery will. Why? Because your body has experienced both and remembers that the chocolate cake is more calorically dense and thus has more survival value. Dopamine drives desire for the chocolate cake through a survival-based capacity known as *attentional bias*, meaning you're going to pay extra attention to the more rewarding stimuli at the expense of other less important, neutral stimuli.[39] Think of it as a big red arrow that flashes in your mind to focus on the most salient (*significant*) stimuli—in this case, chocolate cake. This survival mechanism is essential, yet this is also how we get hooked. Back to the berries in the woods: when you're hungry and you see the berries overhead, dopamine is released to help you focus on obtaining the berries so you don't get easily distracted by your surroundings—and unintentionally die of starvation.

Dopamine dishes out a double whammy. We see the chocolate cake and dopamine is released. We feel pleasure, and we become more focused on the chocolate cake. This is how we get hooked in a loop, sometimes making it hard to focus on anything other than that chocolate cake. The more you think about it, the more you get sucked into its force field. You have a bite and it's all over. Fireworks are going off in your brain, including a rush of dopamine that brings hyper-pleasure, and also focuses your attention on the most salient stimuli, which happens to be that piece of cake sitting right in front of you. That's why it's hard to just have one bite, and we usually eat to the point of nausea or until it's all gone.

The best way to break free from this loop is put down the fork and slowly back away from the cake, turn around, and focus on something else. Put your shoes on and go for a walk, listen to music, call a friend—anything that will naturally boost your feel-good brain chemicals (see chapter 10) and will simultaneously focus your attention elsewhere, like on your long-term goals (see chapter 6).

The Prefrontal Cortex

Unfortunately, when it comes to the negative consequences of dopamine over-stimulation, the story doesn't end here. A study published in 2008 by Dr. Volkow and colleagues revealed a significant negative correlation between BMI and metabolic activity in the prefrontal cortex (PFC).[40] The PFC is the part of the brain associated with higher-order thinking like planning, goal-setting, and mental flexibility, as well as self-monitoring and regulating impulses.[41] It is the most evolved part of our brain and also helps us to resist temptation. These are all tasks related to you saying "no" to that piece of chocolate cake because you want to achieve your long-term health goals. When you flex your PFC, it prevents you from binging on everything in sight because it's part of your rational mind. But the more you give in, the more your dopamine receptor sites decrease or the more your body mass index (BMI, aka weight) increases, the weaker your PFC "muscle" becomes. So not only do you become more hooked on the hyper-palatable foods that excite your taste buds and stimulate your brain, the more you have a harder time saying "no thanks." This also develops into a behavioral pattern that the longer you practice the more difficult it is to reverse (more about habits in chapter 5). Luckily, you can help strengthen your PFC with many of recommendations throughout this book, including exercise, balancing your blood sugar levels with a whole foods diet, meditation, reducing stress, and getting good quality sleep.

Understanding Sugar, Fat, and Salt

Now more than ever, people are confused about what they should eat. Whole food sources of sugar, fat, and sodium are essential to our survival. When eaten in proper ratios from a whole food source, these nutrients in and of themselves are not the problem; they are not evil and you don't have to spend the rest of your days avoiding or hiding from them. But awareness of the way these ingredients are being refined and combined is necessary to unhook yourself from chronic overeating.

Sugar: Refined Carbohydrates Give Carbohydrates a Bad Name

I remember when the Atkins craze hit. People were eating bacon, eggs, and cheeseburgers—minus the bun—like it was going out of style. Many mainstream "low-carb" diets recognize the damage that refined carbohydrates wreak on our health but have inadvertently given all carbohydrates a bad rap. This has added fuel to the fire, leading people astray from the simple, intuitive process of eating real, whole foods because it condemned a whole category of macronutrients that is essential to survival—carbohydrates.

The confusion about carbohydrates has had far-reaching negative consequences to the health and lives of millions of people. The good news is that understanding the truth about carbohydrates is actually very simple and straightforward, and will help you make better choices about what to eat, covered more in depth in chapter 4.

Feeding Our Hungry Cells

Did you know that carbohydrates are the primary fuel source for our cells? Carbohydrates break down into glucose, a simple sugar, and this is the *preferred* source of fuel for our tissues and cells;[42] even the brain uses glucose exclusively to maintain its proper functioning. Before the body can use any of the three macronutrients (carbohydrates, fat, and protein) they must first be converted into glucose.

Carbohydrates are the easiest macronutrient to convert into our primary fuel source, making it the most efficient way to keep the body running smoothly. If we were to completely cut out carbohydrates, something that's possible only for a limited period of time (a major indication that this "low-carb" way of eating is a restrictive *diet* not a *lifestyle*), our bodies would have to work harder and more inefficiently to convert the calories from proteins and fats into simple sugars for our cells. Simple, whole food carbohydrates, on the other hand, were designed to fuel our cells and break down into glucose easily and efficiently. Wouldn't you rather eat a food source that is already easy to digest and designed to give your cells exactly what they need, rather than make your body work a lot harder to convert everything else (fats, proteins, starches) into glucose?

Essentially, our body runs on sugar—so it's not at evil as you might have thought—but as we will see, not all carbohydrates are created equal. There is a major difference between refined and whole food sugars, and the ones you choose to eat can largely affect the state of your health; this is why discretion is required.

Navigating the Sugar Field

Whenever I teach nutrition workshops, I ask the group to call out words that come to mind when I say the word "sugar." The energy in the room shifts. People say things like "bad" or "unhealthy." I hear things like "processed" or "white" or even "fattening" and "addictive." Someone once even said "sneaky."

This proves to me that some major misconceptions about sugar need to be clarified. It's ironic that those who have been led astray the most often are people firmly rooted in the health community. We've been so brainwashed to fear sugar—to fear *carbs*—that we've missed the big picture, and in the process we've labeled some very different foods under one big scary "carbohydrate" umbrella.

Misinformation and disinformation (misleading information deliberately intended to influence public opinion) has led many people to equate highly refined white sugar with sugar found in fruits and vegetables. Sugar found in whole foods is totally different from extracted, refined sugar; it's like the difference between "real" and "fake," yet we use the same term for both. Of course there's going to be confusion about this topic.

People who have been taught to lump the entire carbohydrate category together as "bad" have neglected an entire category of whole foods and are missing out on the health benefits of eating simple sugars found in fruits and vegetables—in my opinion, the optimal fuel source for our bodies. Instead, people are consuming chemical-laden animal products, as well as packaged foods that exclaim "gluten free," "low carb," or "no added sugar," and then wonder why it's still a battle to lose all those excess pounds.

When we say "carbohydrates," we need to be clear on exactly what we are talking about. Two main distinctions need to be made: refined versus whole and simple versus complex.

Refined Versus Whole Carbohydrates

Due to the advent of processed foods, we now need to distinguish whole food carbohydrates from refined carbohydrates—a distinction we would not have had to make less than one hundred years ago.

A refined food, such as white sugar or white flour, has been extracted from its whole food plant source and processed into a more concentrated substance, involving a chemical and/or mechanical process. Through this process, many of the vitamins, minerals, fiber, and water are removed. This fragmentation drastically increases the speed at which these refined foods enter the bloodstream, a striking resemblance to the refinement of whole plants like poppy into heroin or coca leaves into cocaine. Whether it is sugar, cocaine, or heroin, all originate from a plant source and are refined down to a concentrated substance. It is the refinement process that facilitates quicker-than-normal absorption into the bloodstream, triggering various chemical processes in the brain that in turn affect mood and behavior.

We can find examples of these refined simple carbohydrates everywhere we look, stocking the shelves of every grocery store, including "health food" stores. They include cookies, pastries, ice cream, donuts, candy and chocolate, white breads, table sugar, and refined complex carbohydrates like pastas, pizza, and cereal. They also can be found in most commercially sold beverages. The vast majority of packaged food products include refined sugar. Even supposed "health foods" and "organic treats" are loaded with refined, processed carbohydrates.

According to the World Health Organization, sugars and other refined simple carbohydrates are a leading factor in the worldwide obesity epidemic. Overconsumption of refined sugar, high-fructose corn syrup, and other highly refined carbohydrates has been associated with a higher incidence of obesity,[43] diabetes,[44] coronary heart disease,[45] Crohn's disease,[46] and even breast[47] and colorectal cancer.[48]

Eating disorders including binge eating disorder and bulimia nervosa are also related to overconsumption of high fat and refined carbohydrates.[49]

Whole food, simple carbohydrates are quite different than their refined counterparts. Whole food simple carbohydrates are found in fruits and vegetables and come in their "complete package," which includes the right proportion of water and fiber to help facilitate the natural rate of digestion and absorption. These whole foods have been recognized by every major health organization as promoters of health and wellness, compared to their refined counterparts, promoters of disease and obesity.

Complex Versus Simple Carbohydrates

Besides being whole or refined, carbohydrates are either simple or complex. Simple carbohydrates are either a single sugar molecule or two sugar molecules that have joined together. Because simple carbohydrates consist of one or two sugar molecules, due to their simple structure, they can quickly and easily be broken down into glucose and converted into energy soon after they have been consumed.

Complex carbohydrates are comprised of many sugar molecules, joined together in a chain. They do not taste sweet and are highly unpalatable on their own, unless, of course, you add sugar, fat, and salt. Due to the more complex chemical structure, these particular carbohydrates require a lot more energy to digest than simple carbohydrates and are not broken down as easily. Complex carbohydrates are also known as starches and can be found in grains such as rice and wheat, corn, cereals, roots and tubers like potatoes, bread, pasta, and legumes like beans, peas, and lentils.

Not surprisingly, there is controversy surrounding grains as a health food, with the government promoting it as such. After all, most grains are government-subsidized products, and the products that tend to sell the best are those that are the most heavily advertised. In the next chapter, we will discuss grains more in depth and how they may be contributing to keeping you physiologically hooked.

Fat: A Built-in Preference for More

To ensure the survival of our species, Mother Nature cleverly provided us with a built-in preference for *more* calories as opposed to less. This was a way to ensure we would survive times of famine: eat as much as you can now in case you won't be eating again for who knows how long. We've also been physiologically designed to want more calories as opposed to fewer calories, and when it comes to calories, fat takes the cake. Fat offers us an ultra-sensory experience because it packs more than twice as many calories (9 cal per gram) as protein and carbohydrates (4 cal per gram), which means that when we are exposed to high-fat foods, we tend to overeat.

In our current food environment, we have easy access to fat in many forms, which we now know is quite damaging to our health for many reasons, including the damage it can do to the brain, promoting none other than *further weight gain*. The hypothalamus is the part of the brain that is responsible for certain metabolic processes, including hunger control and regulation. In one study,[50] researchers found that within just twenty-four hours of feeding rats a high-fat diet, their hypothalamus showed increased inflammation, and within one week there was permanent neuron injury. Similar results were found in obese humans. This inflammation of the hypothalamus contributes to leptin resistance (a hunger hormone that inhibits appetite), consequently leading to weight gain.

Fat, Sugar, and Blood Sugar

Fat takes longer to digest than proteins or carbohydrates. When we consume too much fat, it creates a thin coating of fat around the cells, the insulin, and insulin receptor sites, and even blood sugar and the blood vessel walls.[51] This excess fat in the bloodstream prevents the proper uptake of glucose (sugar) from the bloodstream into the cells. When this happens, instead of glucose normally going from bloodstream to cells with the help of insulin (the hormone produced by the pancreas that helps escort glucose into the cells), glucose gets trapped in the bloodstream for longer, which results in sustained, elevated blood sugar levels* and may play a role in other diseases like candidiasis, type II diabetes, and chronic fatigue.

I used to struggle with hypoglycemia, also known as low blood sugar. I remember that once, when I was a child, I stood up to walk across the kitchen, and all of a sudden, I passed out cold on the kitchen floor. That was the first of many fainting experiences, until I learned that I better lie down before I fall down! There's no doubt that eating refined foods can cause blood sugar disorders, especially because they're typically high in fat and refined sugar. When we eat whole foods in their unadulterated states, our bodies process and digest them very differently than they do the refined substance, facilitating the quicker-than-normal absorption into the bloodstream and affecting the stability of blood sugar levels. Couple this with a high dose of fat, as is the case with hyper-palatable foods, and what you have is a sugar party in your bloodstream (hyperglycemia equals high blood sugar). When

---

* For a more thorough explanation of the role of fats, please refer to Dr. Douglas Graham's book "The 80/10/10 Diet"

your brain signals your pancreas to kick into high gear to produce insulin to get all that sugar into your cells, which it eventually does, that's when you feel the "crash" (hypoglycemia equals low blood sugar). You "crash" because an excess of insulin was released while there was too much fat in the bloodstream, and, now that the fat has cleared, the excessive quantity of insulin took too much blood sugar to the cells. What we want are stable blood sugar levels, as these wild fluctuations are contributing factors in both obesity and type II diabetes.

The consequences of hypothalamus inflammation and fluctuating blood sugar levels, combined with unhealthy habitual patterns, stress, emotional eating, and environmental cues, can all contribute to keeping you hooked on hyper-palatable foods, most of which are extremely high in fat.

If weight loss is a part of your goal, then cutting down on fat may be something worth considering. As we will discuss in chapter 4, this is easy to do when you increase your intake of fruits and vegetables. As you make the shift to preparing more of your own meals at home with whole foods, you can avoid the extreme combinations of sugar, fat, and salt that trick you into eating more. Eating a plant-based diet and following the guidelines on limiting fat intake in chapter 4 will help you avoid excess fat, limit your overall calories, and still get all the essential fatty acids that you need.

Salt: Questioning Conventional Thought

Although sodium is essential for life, the question is, "How *much* sodium do you need for optimal health?" Like most people in the health and wellness community, I was taught that salt was good for me. All those nice expensive packages of pink Himalayan crystal salt, Celtic sea salt, and Hawaiian red salt—they all taste so good. But, apparently, a little *too* good.

What Is the Difference between Sodium and Salt?

Although the words "sodium" and "salt" may often be used interchangeably, they are not exactly the same thing. Salt is sodium chloride—about 40 percent sodium and 60 percent chloride.

Sodium is essential to the proper functioning of our bodies, and so is chloride; they are both essential minerals and electrolytes. As we will discuss, we receive these minerals in adequate quantities by eating plant foods. The extracted and concentrated sodium chloride (salt) that we've become habituated to adding to our every meal is not only unnecessary, but hinders proper body functions.

Why Is Excess Sodium Not Ideal?

Our body does not need added salt or sodium.[52] Far more problems result from excess sodium and salt consumption than from not enough. Consider these findings from the Center for Disease Control (CDC):

- As sodium increases, so does blood pressure.
- One in three Americans (nearly 68 million people in the US alone) has high blood pressure.
- High blood pressure is directly linked to an increased risk for heart disease and stroke. (Cardiovascular disease is the leading cause of death in the US.)
- "If all Americans followed the recommended limits for sodium, national rates for high blood pressure would drop by a quarter, saving tens of thousands of lives each year." [53]

Lost at Sea: An Intuitive Perspective

Luckily, there is a very simple, concise explanation about the health-damaging (yes, you read it right) effects of salt in the body. If you were lost at sea, with no fresh water or food, you wouldn't survive very long. If you started to drink seawater to ward off dehydration, you'd be a goner even quicker. What do we all know about drinking seawater? It dehydrates you. And why does it do that? *Because of the salt content.* This isn't any new information, but in fact is quite common knowledge. Now imagine evaporating all the water from saltwater, extracting all the salt, and then eating the very substance that was dehydrating you. What do you think it will do in its now more potent and concentrated form? You guessed it—it's going to dehydrate you. Many people are taught that they should consume salt when they are dehydrated to retain water. Can you see how this is actually terrible advice, only dehydrating the body further?

Sodium and Potassium: A Match Made in Heaven

Considering that the role of sodium in the body is symbiotic with the role of potassium, and how they operate in relation to one another, it would be more appropriate to look at these minerals together. In "primitive" cultures the potassium intake is about seven times higher than sodium intake, which is thought to be optimal.[54] The alarming news is that most people in today's culture are eating far more sodium than potassium—about three times more.

> **Primitive Cultures—Potassium-to-Sodium Ratio: 7:1**
>
> **Developed Cultures—Potassium-to-Sodium Ratio: 1:3**

Why does this matter? Actually, it matters quite a lot. The appropriate ratio of sodium and potassium are critical to the proper functioning of your body. It influences many essential processes, including:

- Helping the nerves and muscles function
- Regulating fluid balance in the body
- Maintaining blood pressure
- Helping control acid-base (pH) balance
- Helping the kidneys function properly
- Serving as cofactors for enzymes in carbohydrate metabolism
- Enabling the transmission of nerve impulses that power the contraction of muscles, including the heart

How Much Sodium and Potassium Do We Really Need?

The so-called official guidelines are confusing, which is inevitable when big business and money are involved. According to the Food and Nutrition Board, under normal conditions the minimal amount of sodium required to replace losses is estimated to be less than 180 mg day,[55] and it recommends a minimum of 500 mg in total per day for those over eighteen. However, the American Heart Association states that we require 1,500 mg daily.[56]

The Report of the Dietary Guidelines Advisory Committee for Americans[57] (which is part of the US Department of Agriculture and their subsequent lobby groups) recommends a *maximum* of 2,300 mg of sodium a day, almost 14 times what our body needs to replace losses. The news gets worse. The average American (over the age of two) consumes a whopping 3,400 milligrams daily[58]—far higher than what our body needs and more than twice the recommended limit for many people. This is an average, which means that some people are consuming even higher quantities of sodium. In this case more is not better, it's worse, and it's wreaking havoc on our health.

The dietary guidelines also recommend that the 70 percent of adults at high risk of sodium-induced illness (people ages fifty-plus, all African Americans, and everyone with high blood pressure, diabetes, or chronic kidney disease) consume fewer than 1,500 mg of sodium per day. Shouldn't that same guidance go for everyone to prevent these diseases in the first place?

About 90 percent of the sodium consumed in the average diet is in excess of bodily needs and is eliminated in the urine.[59] Unfortunately, this also removes potassium from the body, which in turn creates a potassium deficit.

It's quite a different story for potassium; instead of too much, we're not getting enough. The average American consumes about 2,500 mg of potassium a day, about half the 4,700 mg minimum recommended requirements.

Off the Hook

It should be clear that telling someone to just "cut back a little" on refined foods that are highly addictive is like telling a heroin addict to "just say no" to drugs. No one wants to be obese and struggling with food, but without help and addressing the problem for what it actually is—an addiction to refined food—few are capable of making the dietary changes that lead to long-lasting foundational change.

Because the majority of the population eats this way, stepping off this path and onto a new healthier path that revolves around eating abundant amounts of fresh fruits and vegetables is viewed as "being crazy," but isn't our current state of health actually what's crazy?

You can learn to physically unhook yourself from the food struggle by learning to eat real, whole foods. This is how we not only improve an unhealthy relationship with food, but also improve our physical, emotional, psychological, and spiritual well-being.

Are you ready to step into a new paradigm? Are you ready to live in a reality where thoughts of food do not consume the days, weeks, and months of your life? A reality where you no longer experience cravings, addiction, and mood swings and where the majority of your days are no longer rooted in feelings of fear, guilt, shame, suffering, compulsion, and obsession, but instead you feel stable, balanced, and even joyful?

Only you can take this step. No one else can take it for you. *Are you ready?*

Chapter 4

Unhooked: Transitioning to a Whole Foods Lifestyle

Shifting towards a whole foods lifestyle can take some getting used to as you adjust and learn to navigate your way through our current food environment. By now, you're starting to see that many of the food products sold in grocery stores are actually food imitations: food impostors standing in for the real deal. Now you might be wondering, how do I transition to whole foods; what do I eat?

Welcome to the wonderful world of *real, whole food*. This requires a welcomed shift away from processed, packaged foods toward vibrant, colorful, real foods. Understandably, there will always be a debate when it comes to nutrition-specific recommendations. Some people may question the dietary recommendations outlined in this chapter. If you notice yourself becoming defensive or upset by my proposed solutions, this may be opportunity to explore your food-related belief systems. Keep in mind that what's presented in this chapter are only concepts and ideas that I believe to be true—based on years of personal experimentation and professional study. We are all travelers on our own personal journeys of discovery. I encourage you to explore, experiment, and question the concepts presented to discover what is true for you, as I have done for myself. These eight recommendations have helped me enormously, and provide you with the opportunity to learn how I became unhooked from years of food addiction, disordered eating, and fluctuating weight levels. Following these guidelines has allowed me to break free from this struggle, and so I offer them here for you to take into consideration on your own journey.

If you do choose to implement the suggestions in this chapter, remember that it can take time to firmly root yourself in a new routine, and it can have its challenging moments, especially where family and friends are concerned. But what's worse: living with discontent in your body, mind, and spirit, or stepping into a new way of living that might have a bit of a learning curve? What do you have to lose? If you don't like it, I can assure you that processed foods will always be there for you to go back to. But you may be surprised that once you really know how good it feels to, well . . . feel good, you won't want to be running back to the standard American diet (SAD) way of living any time soon.

Following these guidelines can help you restore homeostasis and prevent your hedonic pleasure drive from taking over. It's important to choose foods that don't "artificially" overstimulate you or deplete your dopamine receptor sites, so that you can gain greater enjoyment from the positive, health-affirming pleasures in life, like walking in the park, spending time with your children, and enjoying the (non-addictive) satisfaction of eating real, whole food.

Two Things We Know for Sure

Despite all the confusion and contradictory information about the hundreds (maybe even thousands) of diets, there are two things that we know for sure: that the Western diet is disease promoting, and fruits and vegetables are health promoting.

Without getting mired in the microscopic details of individual nutrients, on a broader scale, we know that the standard American diet (SAD), also referred to as a Western diet, is causing us more harm than good. No one is arguing this point. Not long after other cultures around the world adopt the SAD lifestyle, they also develop the same diseases that are running rampant in our culture, including obesity, type II diabetes, cancer, and cardiovascular disease, to name a few. This diet consists of large amounts of factory-farmed animal products, processed foods, refined sugar, and refined grains, with large amounts of fat and too much salt. It is also a diet of *too much* of everything *except* whole, fresh fruits and vegetables.

There is consensus within the medical community that fruits and vegetables are health promoting, and they should be an integral part of a healthy diet. We don't need to focus on which particular fruit or vegetable has which particular miraculous nutrient: we just need to consume a wide variety of them in abundant quantities. With this in mind, fruits and vegetables take center stage in a real, whole foods lifestyle.

There are many reasons why eating a diet predominated by fruits and vegetables is a good idea, and one of those reasons has to do with willpower. Research suggests that maintaining stable blood sugar levels play an important role in self-control.[60] And guess what? This real, whole foods dietary lifestyle helps to maintain stable blood sugar levels, reduce impulsivity, and gives you a little willpower boost to help you steer clear of packaged, processed foods. Eating this way will also help prevent a wide range of diseases, help you lose weight, and unhook you from the addictive qualities of foods that comprise the SAD lifestyle. This is how we go from SAD to happy . . . and free from the food struggle.

"Fruits and vegetables are the one point of consensus—an oasis—in arguments about what to eat. Everyone agrees that eating more of them is a good idea."

—**Marion Nestle,** *What to Eat*

A Word about Transitioning

Before we discuss the guidelines outlined in this chapter, it's worth taking a moment to talk about *transitioning* to a healthier lifestyle. This is usually the heart of what everyone wants to know—*how* to transition, what concrete steps to take to feel better, lose weight, and get healthier.

These are valid questions, and the answer is: it depends on you. I will provide guidance and suggestions, but it will be up to you to decide how fast you want to make the shift and what initial steps you can take that will work best for you in particular. You have to go at your own pace and do what genuinely *feels good* for you, otherwise you may set yourself up for a major backlash (I'm sure you're familiar with the phrase "off the wagon"), and this is not what we are going for.

Transitioning depends on your personality. Some people like to dive right in; other people like to take it one small incremental step at a time. Whatever your approach, there are seven simple principles to keep in mind:

1. **This is not a diet; this is a lifestyle.** This way of eating is a long-term, sustainable way to live. Being healthy is not only about food; it's about

staying active, doing the work you love, maintaining a positive outlook on life, and following all the other lifestyle-oriented recommendations throughout this book to give you a daily dose of those feel-good chemicals in your brain.

2. **This is not about deprivation; this is a lifestyle of abundance.** Trying to lose weight through deprivation does not work, plain and simple. That's why I love eating mostly fruits and vegetables, because as you will see, you can eat as much as you want of these low-calorie yet nutrient-dense whole foods.

3. **Slow and steady wins the race (not that this is a race).** We need to let go of the notion that we can "lose 7 pounds in 7 days." This is not a quick-fix solution. It's more important to become aware of the direction you're headed in rather than on how fast you get there. This also means letting go of an all-or-nothing mentality and not giving up all hope in the face of a small slip-up.

4. **Difficult transitioning is largely a mental barrier.** Transitioning to a whole foods lifestyle is fortunately much easier than most people believe. The biggest hurdle to overcome is the mental barrier to transitioning. Frame your transition in whatever way makes the most logical sense in your mind to help support you in this journey. Remember: you don't have to (and it's better if you don't) put yourself in a mentally constructed and rigidly defined "dietary box"; this is only more likely to set you up for failure.

5. **Step out of an all-or-nothing mentality.** Most people tend to think in extremes, especially when it comes to diet. I advocate a diet *predominated* by fruits and vegetables, not *only* of fruits and vegetables. I choose to eat this way because it genuinely makes me happy and it freed me from food addiction. But there is a fine line between following a way of eating and taking it to the extreme that brings only anxiety and guilt when you can't live up to unrealistic expectations. Being happy (genuine long-term happiness, not the fleeting pleasurable "happiness" we seek in hyper-palatable food) is imperative to your long-term success in following a healthy diet and lifestyle.

6. **This is a path, not a destination.** When it comes to transitioning, it's important to remember that we are *always in transition*. It is a continuous journey, an unfolding process. Despite what we've determined as the

"destination," we never really get "there" because there is no "there." We can always take another step, however small, in the direction of better health and well-being. And if you're dedicated to this, this will become a fun and joyful lifelong path, one that brings many benefits. It's not about striving, but rather staying steadfast on your journey, with each step taking you towards better health.

7. **Focus on what you can have, not on what you can't.** When I coach my clients on how to transition, there is a strong emphasis on what to include—what you *can* eat—and less emphasis on what you should avoid eating. The more you eat fresh fruits and vegetables, the more you naturally have less room for everything else. Simply start by focusing on the foods you want to include rather than the foods you're looking to remove.

Unhook Yourself by Learning What to Eat

These two very simple facts—that the SAD leads to an early grave and that a plant-based diet consisting of mostly fruits and vegetables prevents disease and promotes longevity—along with years of research, experimenting with my own diet, and working with clients on transitioning to healthier lifestyles, made me realize that choosing *what* to eat is actually a lot simpler than originally thought. If you're ready to start aligning with the nourishment your body was designed to receive and reap the major benefits that go along with it, follow these seven simple guidelines:

1. Eat real, whole food
2. Eat food in simple combinations
3. Eat mostly fruits and vegetables
4. Reduce consumption of animal products
5. Reduce fat intake to 10-15 percent of total calories
6. Work towards eliminating salt intake
7. Choose your grains wisely, if you must eat them at all

Following these eight simple guidelines allows you to eat in a way that mirrors nature and most closely matches your physiological needs, despite living in an unnatural food environment. This is the basis of how to end the internal struggle with food, let go of food addiction, lose weight, prevent disease, and reclaim your health.

1. Eat Real, Whole Food

Let's come back to square one: we know that foods from the earth are what our bodies were designed to eat, not the synthetic products that "food science" has so cleverly concocted. When you're wondering if a food is a real, whole food or not, simply ask yourself, "Can I find this in nature?"

Here are the top-six criteria for healthy plant-based food:[61]

1. Whole
2. Fresh
3. Ripe
4. Raw
5. Organic
6. Local

These are just guidelines; you don't have to eat only foods that fit all six criteria (remember, we're letting go of all-or-nothing thinking), although the more you eat of these foods, the more you (and the environment) will benefit. Even though most of my diet consists of raw food, I was hesitant to include the "raw" criterion to avoid the "raw versus cooked" debate. This is not a book about transitioning to a raw food lifestyle. Having said that, everyone can benefit from increasing their intake of raw fruits and vegetables. This doesn't mean that you have to eat *only* raw foods, but increasing your intake of raw fruits and vegetables is a good place to start. This doesn't mean you can never eat cooked pumpkin soup or sautéed mushrooms or grilled eggplant ever again; just try to eat more foods that fall within the six criteria. Essentially, pursue the simple pleasures of raw fruits and vegetables and all of the wonderfully delicious ways to combine them to create decadent, nourishing, tasty meals.

Avoid packaged food products. When you start to eat foods in their natural state, the need for packaged items naturally becomes less frequent. When you eat from a package it means that someone else has done some level of processing to the food, making it one more step removed from nature. It also means that the package contributes to waste, making it an unsustainable long-term alternative to nature's own "packaging." At this point I invite you to start noticing how often you reach for packaged foods.

If you are buying packaged foods, read the label. I know that completely giving up packaged foods is challenging and may take some time to transition.

When you do buy packaged foods, be sure to read the labels and try to follow these general guidelines:

- Avoid products with a long list of ingredients.
- Avoid products with ingredients you can't pronounce and don't recognize—if you can't recognize it, your body probably can't either.
- Avoid products with wheat, soy, corn, and refined sugar (be careful, as these are disguised under very many different and obscure names).
- Avoid products that contain cheap oils like soybean, canola, or vegetable oils.

2. Eat Food in Simple Combinations

When we were forced to forage for food, it was highly unlikely that we would put together five or six dishes, containing upwards of dozens of ingredients, and sit down for a picnic. Thanks to the industrial food revolution, this is a relatively new phenomenon.

Remember that fat or sugar on its own produces a less intense experience for the brain than when combined. We discussed in chapter 3 that taste is hardwired to our pleasure center and that these complex tastes excite and stimulate the brain. When the brain fires more (rather than less) electrical signals, it means we want it more (whatever food we're seeing, tasting, smelling, or hearing) and then tend to eat to excess. Returning to simple food combinations will satisfy you without the hyper-stimulation. We also discussed in chapter 1 that food variety can lead to overconsumption, so scratch the all-you-can-eat buffets, even healthy ones, off your list. Eating many foods in one sitting can also cause you digestive upset, while eating simple food combinations are easier on your digestive system. This makes a strong case for simplifying meals. When making a meal, try limiting your ingredients to four to five foods. Also be mindful that even "health" food companies use extreme food combinations to get people to like their foods and favor their products, albeit perhaps with better quality ingredients.

3. Eat Mostly Fruits and Vegetables

Every major health organization, including the World Health Organization, the American Medical Association, the American Diabetes Association, and the American Cancer Society, recognizes the health benefits of fruits and vegetables as an important part of a healthy diet. Eating fresh fruits and vegetables is associated with the prevention of a wide range of diseases,[62] including cancer (bladder, breast, cervical, colorectal, esophageal, kidney, lung, ovarian, pancreatic, prostate, and stomach),[63] cardiovascular disease[64] (coronary heart disease[65] and stroke), type II diabetes,[66] and obesity.[67]

"Fruit comes in an intricate, highly nutritious package that matches our nutritional needs better than any other category of food. I recommend that virtually our entire carbohydrate intake—80 percent of calories or more—come from the simple sugars in whole, fresh fruit."

—Dr. Douglas Graham, *The 80/10/10 Diet*

Despite fruit being recognized as a health food from every health-related organization, there's still much confusion surrounding this incredibly important food group. There's less disagreement over whether vegetables should take center stage in our diets, but fruit tends to be criticized more often because of the whole misconception of sugar and carbohydrates discussed in chapter 3. The health benefits of whole fruits and vegetables is one of the very few things that we know for sure, yet there are still "health" professionals advising people to steer clear of fruit because of all the "sugar." But as we saw, whole food sugars are quite different from processed and refined sugars and act very differently in the body.

The Miracle of Fruits and Vegetables

Fruits and vegetables are the most *nutrient-dense* foods on the planet. In addition to being low in calories, mostly low in saturated fat (coconut and avocado are two exceptions), and containing only trace amounts of cholesterol, these two incredible food groups take either the #1 or #2 position regarding our most essential nutrient needs. When fruits come in first, vegetables come in second, and vice versa. Combined, fruits and vegetables are our absolute best sources of:

- Water
- Fiber
- Vitamins
- Minerals
- Phytonutrients
- Antioxidants
- Fructose and glucose

- Enzymes and co-enzymes
- Guar and pectin (two soluble fibers that slow sugar uptake)

Since fruits and vegetables take the #1 and #2 spots in meeting our nutritional requirements, they should comprise the bulk of the foods you consume. Eating a varied fruit- and vegetable-based diet also naturally provides you with the optimal caloric-nutrient ratio of carbohydrates, proteins, and fats to satisfy your body's requirements.

I know many people who removed fruit from their diets because they were afraid it would cause blood sugar disorders like hyper- and hypoglycemia, type II diabetes, and candidiasis. Even I was surprised to discover that it's not the fruit that is causing the problem. Fruit comes in a total package complete with everything it needs to deliver the sugar to our cells in the most optimal way possible.

The best part about eating a diet primarily of fruits and vegetables is that it has a built-in self-regulating system: water and fiber. These two very important nutrients prevent us from overeating simply because they significantly increase the volume of these foods, promoting satiety. Water and fiber also regulate the efficient transition of the sugar into our bloodstream and then into our cells by preventing the natural sugars from being released too quickly in the bloodstream. It does this more slowly than when eating refined sugar, but quickly enough to easily integrate into our bodies. This provides our cells with an optimal fuel source with minimal energy required by our bodies to digest.

The removal of fiber during the juicing process is one reason why some health experts don't recommend juicing, which is a valid point because fruit juices can also spike blood sugar levels. I do, however, recommend fresh fruit juices over store-bought artificial ones—remember, it's about taking steps in the right direction. Due to the lower simple sugar content in vegetables, "green" juices don't pose the same blood sugar risk and offer a healthy dose of vitamins, minerals, and water. Juicing can definitely be considered one of the "grey" areas I was referring to in chapter 1, because once you remove the fiber, it's technically not a whole food. This is where you have to use your best judgment. I personally really enjoy incorporating fresh vegetable juices into my life. Although I do recommend whole, fresh foods over juices, in certain cases juicing can play an important role, especially during transitioning to a healthier lifestyle. I've seen many people (myself included) benefit from "green" juices, which are juices that are predominantly vegetable based and have little or minimal added juice from fruits.

The high water and fiber content is one of the primary reasons fruits and vegetables are relatively low-calorie foods, making this an ideal dietary lifestyle for maintaining optimal weight levels. You can essentially sit down and eat all the fruit and vegetables you care for and still be able to lose weight because by the time you're full, you've still consumed less calories than eating processed foods that are high in refined sugar, fat, and salt that are not only calorically dense but that trick you into overeating. Compared to the SAD, eating a high fruit and vegetable diet is a higher volume diet. That's why you can save your big plates for your fruit- and vegetable-based meals, as mentioned in chapter 2, and use small plates for cooked food. This higher volume simply means you take more bites in a day to get the necessary calories you need to maintain normal weight levels, and I know some of you are very happy to hear that. That's what makes this a lifestyle of *abundance*, not *deprivation*. You can eat all the fruits and veggies you want to and simply allow your body to take care of the rest.

" . . . the speed at which sugar enters the blood is not really the most important factor. When fruits are eaten whole, with their fiber intact, as part of a low-fat diet, their sugars do indeed enter the bloodstream relatively quickly. But then they also exit just as quickly, making them the ideal food, one that provides the perfect fuel for human consumption."

—**Dr. Douglas Graham,** *The 80/10/10 Diet*

Fruit contains lower levels of sugar than most people think and doesn't spike blood sugar levels like most have been led to believe, unless in the presence of unnaturally high levels of fat (more about this shortly). There is a common myth that fruits are all high-glycemic foods, which means they spike insulin levels (which is not a good thing), but this is incorrect. Please refer to Appendix B for more information on fruit and the glycemic index.

Some Tips to Get You Started
Start drinking green smoothies. In case you haven't noticed, there is a green smoothie revolution taking place. Is it happening in your kitchen yet? I cannot overemphasize how pivotal this one dietary change can be to your lifestyle. If you're not sure how to increase your consumption of fruits and vegetables, start with smoothies. Try replacing either your breakfast or lunch with a fruit or

vegetable-based smoothie. Here are a couple of my favorite recipes that you can enjoy as a meal:

Blueberry Blast

2 cups fresh or frozen organic blueberries

3 organic fresh or frozen bananas

2 packed cups organic spinach

1 cup coconut water or purified water

Mango Love

2 cups fresh or frozen organic mango

3 organic fresh or frozen bananas

½ bunch of organic kale

1 cup coconut water or purified water

Pear Cilantro Deliciousness

3 organic medium sized pear

3 fresh or frozen organic banana

1 bunch cilantro

1 date

Morning Detox Smoothie

1 medium-sized organic cucumber

3 fresh or frozen organic bananas

1 tablespoon spirulina powder

1 cup coconut water or purified water

With smoothies, you can essentially blend up whatever fruit or vegetables you have. A winning smoothie recipe usually involves:

Any sweet fruit + banana + leafy green + coconut water ovr regular water

Avoid using fruit juices in your smoothies; your smoothies will be sweet enough from the whole, raw fruits you use. Also, you may want to work your way up to the taste of "green." If you've been eating a SAD for many years, it can take a little bit of time to rewire your taste buds to prefer natural over artificial tastes. This happens relatively fast, as your taste buds regenerate quickly, approximately every three weeks, providing you with the opportunity to acquire the taste (and the love) of whole foods.

Try new fruits and vegetables. People tend to buy the same fruits and vegetables repeatedly, as we are creatures of habit. Instead, try something new; try one new fruit or vegetable every week and expose your palate to new flavors and textures.

Explore the colors of the rainbow. All the different phytonutrients (plant chemicals) have a wide range of health benefits. When you're exploring your produce section, intuitively pick the colors that attract you.

Have fun with new recipes. Get creative and dive in! If buying mostly fresh fruits and vegetables is new to you, have fun with it. Look up new recipes online, experiment with new ideas, and create meals that taste good to you. Check out my website www.happyandraw.com for a whole slew of healthy fruit- and vegetable-based recipes you can make at home.

Shop the periphery of the store. When grocery shopping, spend more of your time in the produce section. Fresh foods are always sold along the periphery of the store. Notice how much food you normally buy from the entire middle section of the grocery store and try to avoid all middle aisles whenever possible.

Find local produce. A great way to find local, organic fruits and vegetables is to check out your local farmers markets, join an organic food co-operative, or sign up for a fruit and vegetable delivery service like CSA (Community Supported Agriculture). CSAs either have a drop spot where you can pick up fresh, whole foods every week, and some even deliver right to your home.

4. Reduce Consumption of Animal Products

There is always going to be a debate about whether we should or shouldn't consume animal products. I personally choose to not include any meat or dairy products in my diet for a wide range of reasons, but could I honestly say without a shadow of a doubt that this is the best choice for *everyone*? No, I can't. But there are some really good reasons why you may want to consider steering clear of these foods, or at least experiment with reducing your consumption.

If you haven't yet read the book *The China Study* by T. Colin Campbell, I highly recommend you do. Through a comprehensive study, involving 6,500 men and women from 65 counties in China, a very strong correlation between meat, dairy, and egg consumption and cancer was found; the higher the meat consumption, the greater the risk of cancer. And not just for one kind of cancer, but for a wide range of diseases, including cancer of the colon, lung, breast, prostate, stomach, and liver, as well as an increased risk of obesity, osteoporosis, autoimmune diseases, diabetes, rheumatoid arthritis, kidney stones, dementia, Alzheimer's, and heart disease.[68]

Dr. Campbell is not alone in studying the link between meat consumption and the development of cancer. Meat consumption in relation to cancer risk has been reported in over a hundred epidemiological studies from many countries with diverse diets.[69] The National Institute of Health (NIH) Diet and Health Study studied approximately 500,000 men and women in the United States, among whom over 53,000 incident cancers occurred. The study showed that the consumption of red meat increased the risk of esophagus, liver, and lung cancer between 20 to 60 percent. Other findings include: a 16 percent increased risk of lung cancer related to the consumption of processed meats, a 24 percent increased risk in colorectal cancer with red meat consumption, and a 20 percent increased risk with processed meat consumption.[70]

Contrary to fruits and vegetables, meat and dairy products are high in calories, saturated fat, cholesterol, antibiotics, and growth hormones; contain potentially carcinogenic compounds including nitrosamines, nitrosamides and heterocyclic amines; are acidifying to the body; low in water, vitamins, and minerals; and contain no fiber or carbohydrates. People also tend to eat meat in combination with refined sugars, fat, and salt, as meat is largely unpalatable on its own.

Whether or not we are meant to be omnivores from purely a health-centric perspective, we also still need to take into consideration the impact that these foods have on our environment. Many books have been written about the environmental devastation caused by meat consumption so I won't go into detail here, except to mention that factory farming is a major polluter, to say the least. We need to consider the bigger picture and not only what *our* needs are, but look at the greater impact these industries are having on our environment, our water supply, and biodiversity, not to mention the extremely inhumane living conditions for millions of animals. This alone is enough of a reason to seriously consider cutting back on animal products.

Hooked on Cheese

I've lost track of how many times I've heard clients confess the inability to stop consuming cheese. It seems to be one of the last high-fat foods that people are willing to give up. I completely empathize; I was once a cheese addict too, and sometimes I still feel the hidden lure of this particular food.

Neal Barnard, MD, author of *Breaking the Food Seduction* and president of the Physicians Committee for Responsible Medicine, explains that the addictive quality of these dairy products is due to the small amounts of morphine (an addictive opiate) in the cow's milk as well as a protein called casein. Casein breaks apart during digestion to release a whole host of opiates called casomorphins. These stimulate those "feel-good" brain chemicals that we've been talking about and drive our craving for the foods that contain these casomorphins. A cup of cow's milk contains about six grams of casein, and cheese contains far more, as one pound of cheese contains about ten pounds of milk. As milk is turned into cheese, most of its water, whey proteins, and lactose sugar are removed, leaving behind concentrated casein and fat, delivering a whopping 400 calories in 100 grams of a standard cheddar cheese.

In his book, Dr. Campbell suggests a protein intake of no higher than 10 percent of total calories and suggests that based on his findings, consuming more than that places us at increased risk for getting cancer. He also goes on to say: "For all these experiments, we were using casein, which makes up 87 percent of cow's milk protein. So the next logical question was whether plant protein, tested in the same way, has the same effect on cancer promotion as casein. The answer is an astonishing NO. *In these experiments, plant protein did not promote cancer growth, even at higher levels of intake.*"[71]

"In our society, protein deficiency is practically nonexistent. Instead, most people consume too much protein, which can also affect health adversely . . . Cutting down on protein will free up energy, spare your digestive system and especially your liver and kidneys from extra work, and protect your immune system from irritation."

—Andrew Weil, M.D., *Spontaneous Healing*

If You Must . . .

Although I believe that most people can benefit from reducing their intake of animal products, if you do choose to continue to eat animal products, become mindful of your consumption and try to make it a very small portion of your diet. Respect and give thanks for the animal you are about to ingest. I always recommend to people that they should go through their own experience of raising and killing an animal if they wish to consume them. A couple years ago, I watched my husband "harvest" a chicken and prepare it for dinner. It was a very eye-opening experience and confirmed my feeling that meat consumption is not for me. After a more direct "up close and personal" experience with the "harvesting" (which means killing) process, you too may have a different stance on meat consumption. Try to move away from red meat altogether; avoid cured meats, cold cuts, and ground meats. Consume the best "quality" meats you can find, choosing quality over quantity, and experiment with reducing your overall consumption. Follow these general guidelines to consume the best source possible:

- **Grass-fed.** Most of the conventional factory-farming producers feed their animals corn and grain-based feed that is usually low quality and genetically modified. Grass feeding is at least more aligned with their natural diets and usually allows the animals space to roam.
- **Free range.** This is a term only applied to chickens and means that the animals had access to outdoor space, allowing them to move, as opposed to the extremely confined living conditions of factory farms. When the chickens are free range, they typically eat more grass, making their meat more nutritious (eating plants as opposed to grains provides more nutritional value for meat), get more exercise (producing a leaner meat), and get fresh air and sunlight. They also tend to be less stressed (from overcrowding) and experience less disease, reducing the need for antibiotics.
- **Buy organic when you can.** Choosing certified organic meats and dairy will help you to reduce your consumption of antibiotics, pesticides, growth hormones, and genetically modified foods.
- **Go local.** Whenever possible, support a local provider and ask for a tour of their farm to check out farming practices. You will get better quality meats from small, sustainable farms rather than the large, industrial farms.

For those of you who have decided to stop consuming meat products, I highly recommend steering clear of all the fake imitation meat products like "vegan" bacon, pepperoni, and other imitation deli meats. I think the concept of eating *real* food also applies here. One year I went to a "vegetarian" potluck for Thanksgiving and saw my first "fake" vegetarian chicken, which was an interesting mix of gluten, wheat, soy, and chemicals—definitely a result of "food science." If I absolutely had to choose between the two, I would probably opt for the real meat over fake. Luckily I don't have to choose; I can just stick with fruits and vegetables.

When it comes to dairy, consider vegan dairy alternatives (although I don't recommend store-bought, soy-based products). Try homemade nut and seed milks instead; they are great for transitioning to a plant-based diet and are far tastier than any cow's milk I ever tried. They also happen to be healthier, more cost-effective, and take no time at all to make yourself. Check out my website www.happyandraw.com for some simple nut milk recipes.

5. Work Towards Reducing Fat Intake to 10-15 percent of Total Calories

It's easy to get lured into the debate over single nutrients. While deciding what to include in this section, when researching saturated fat I was confronted with a whole slew of contradictory information. I was reminded once again to step back and look at the bigger picture. When the majority of our daily diet consists of the lower-fat fruits and vegetables (most fruits and vegetables are low fat), regardless of what the smaller portion of your diet consists of—*as long as it's real, whole food* (examples include sprouts, leafy greens, and small portions of higher-fat foods like nuts, seeds, avocado, and coconut), you're going to be within the safe zone for total fat intake and definitely within the safe zone for saturated fat intake. The same cannot be said for the SAD lifestyle. When it comes to the SAD, most people are eating too much fat and mostly the wrong kinds.

How Much Fat Do We Need?

The last thing I want to create is a fear of fat. Fat is essential in our diets, especially the essential fatty acids (the omega-3s and 6s). Instead we need to shift our thinking toward an optimal *balance* of the three macronutrients: carbohydrates, proteins, and fats.

All plants contain a percentage of carbohydrates, proteins, and fats—so there's no such thing as a no-fat or no-carb diet that also includes whole plant foods. Many renowned health professionals, including Dr. Douglas Graham, Dr. John McDougall, and Dr. Dean Ornish, advocate a low-fat diet where fat comprises about 10–15 percent of total calories, compared to the 35-40 percent fat intake of the average American.

Luckily, plant foods have insignificant amounts of cholesterol, and most fruits and vegetables are naturally low in fat (especially saturated fat), with anywhere from 2 to 15 percent of calories from fats (there are a few exceptions, including avocado, durian, and coconut). The more you increase your intake of these healthy plant foods, the more your intake of fat will naturally decrease. In fact, a natural diet of fruits and vegetables (especially leafy greens), along with small amounts of a variety of seeds and nuts, avocado, or coconut, provides the body with all the essential fatty acids it needs.

Here are some important guidelines worth considering when it comes to fats:

1. Get your fats through real, whole foods.
2. Choose fresh, raw nuts and seeds.
3. Eat an optimal ratio of omega-3s and 6s.
4. Remember that calories from fats add up fast.
5. Completely avoid trans fats.

A. Get Your Fats through Real, Whole Foods

The concept of eating real, whole foods applies to meeting all of our nutritional needs, including fats. Fats are essential to your body, and you will receive the most benefits if you eat them in their whole food state rather than in a refined state, which includes oils. This is because the fats that are most beneficial (monounsaturated and polyunsaturated) are the most delicate and immediately start to deteriorate once they are extracted from their whole food source.

Refined oils are just that—*refined*. We all know about refined foods, mainly to *avoid them!* The same applies to oils. Just as wheat is stripped of many of its nutrients to make a refined flour product, so too are fats extracted from whole food sources to make a fractional food "product" that is now 100 percent concentrated fat. What we are left with, the real bang for your buck, is what we call *empty calories*—calories from food that supply energy but are nutritionally unbalanced.

Whole foods are a complete package provided by nature to protect the fats from the damaging effects of light, oxygen, and heat, making them less prone to the damaging effects of free radicals. It would be hard to refute that the greatest health benefits from these fats occur when they are consumed in their whole food packages and are extracted and broken down through chewing, as opposed to any kind of machine. It's easy—instead of consuming oil, opt for the whole food instead: flaxseeds rather than flax oil, and hemp seeds rather than hemp oil. The same goes for avocado, macadamia, almond, etc.

As with all foods, we can always take a step in the right direction. I've presented a general scale for oils below ranging from 1 to 4, with 1 being the *least* optimal and 4 being the *most* optimal choice. Wherever you are on the scale, keep working your way up. Avoid cheap vegetable oils and move towards whole food fat sources instead.

1. Vegetable Oils

Do your best to completely avoid vegetable oils, including foods that are made with them. Vegetable oils are usually soy based but also include canola, corn, peanut, and safflower oils. These are cheap oils, sold in clear, plastic bottles and usually stocked in the middle aisles of the grocery store.

2. Olive Oils

1. Olive oil
2. Virgin olive oil
3. Extra virgin olive oil
4. Organic, cold-pressed extra virgin olive oil sold in a dark bottle with a low acidity rating

3. High Omega-3 Oils

1. Walnut oil
2. Hemp oil
3. Udo's DHA 3-6-9 oil blend
4. Flax oil

When purchasing any oils, whether they are the olive oils or any of the "better" quality, high omega-3 oils, make sure to buy cold-pressed, organic oils that come in a dark bottle (light exposure will oxidize the oil faster) and sold in the refrigerated section.

4. Whole Foods

Rather than consuming oils—a 100 percent fat source—opt for whole foods instead. By eating sufficient quantities of fruits and vegetables, you will be consuming enough essential fatty acids to meet your needs in a balanced ratio. The best source of any nutrient is not necessarily the food that has the highest amount of a particular nutrient (how often have you heard: "this food is the highest source of…") but rather that is bundled with the most complete package of balanced nutrition. That being said, there are some excellent "complete package" foods that offer an excellent source of essential fatty acids:

- Flaxseeds
- Chia seeds
- Hemp seeds

- Avocados
- Almonds
- Walnuts
- Sesame (tahini)

B. Choose raw nuts and seeds

When shopping for nuts and seeds, make sure you buy them fresh, organic, and raw. The roasted and salted varieties are detrimental to your health, as they are very high in sodium, and the unstable, delicate fats are more likely to turn rancid from heat exposure. Even packaged raw nuts and seeds can go rancid; that's why fresh is always best. There are many organic raw food suppliers online where you can buy great quality raw nuts and seeds. A simple Google search can help you find a distributor in your area.

C. Eat an Optimal Ratio of Omega-3 to Omega-6

It is very important to consume essential fatty acids, including omega-3 (alpha-linolenic acid, or ALA) and omega-6 (linoleic acid, or LA). They are polyunsaturated fats and are essential because they are vital for human health, as they are precursors for making other required fatty substances that the body can't make on its own; you must get them through food. It's important to eat an optimal ratio of these fats within the range of 1:1 to 4:1 (omega-6 to omega-3).

Omega-3 helps reduce inflammation, and omega-6 promotes inflammation. Although omega-6 is considered to be essential, most people are consuming too much of it, with common sources including safflower, corn, cottonseed, and soybean oils. The average American tends to consume 14–25 times more omega-6 fatty acids than omega-3 fatty acids. This lopsided ratio has been shown to promote many diseases, including cardiovascular disease, cancer, and inflammatory and autoimmune diseases, whereas a more balanced ratio (1:1–5:1) suppressed these effects. [72]

Omega-3 fatty acids are highly concentrated in the brain and implicated in cognitive (brain memory and performance) and behavioral function. A deficiency can lead to fatigue, poor memory, mood swings, and depression, as well as heart problems. Research shows that omega-3 fatty acids reduce inflammation and may help lower risk of chronic diseases such as heart disease, cancer, and arthritis. [73]

When we eat foods high in alpha-linolenic acid (ALA), it is converted into two longer chain omega-3 fatty acids, EPA and DHA, of which fish is the main source.

Some people argue it is best to get EPA and DHA directly from fish instead of eating plant foods high in ALA and risk a low conversion rate to EPA and DHA. This is still largely unknown, but it may be possible that if we consume an optimal ratio of omegas and don't overconsume LA compared to ALA, the conversion rates may be improved. This is because the enzymes that work on them are exactly the same, and if we eat too much LA, it can compete with the enzymes that help convert ALA into EPA and DHA.

While you can choose to get omega-3s from fish (particularly mackerel and salmon, but make sure to find a good quality source), or from fish oil supplements (look for supplements that are tested for mercury levels), I believe the best source of omega-3s is plant foods. The dietary recommendation for ALA is 1.6 grams per day and 1.1 grams per day for men and women respectively, 19 years and older.

Some great plant-based sources of omega-3s include:

- Flaxseed (1 tablespoon has over 1 gram of omega-3, about 140 percent of daily requirement)
- Chia seed (1 ounce of chia seeds has over 5 grams of omega-3, over 450 percent of daily requirement)
- Hemp seed
- Walnuts
- Dark green, leafy vegetables (kale, spinach, salad greens)
- Purslane
- Chickpeas
- Winter squash
- Berries
- Mango
- Jackfruit
- Cauliflower
- Brussel sprouts

Avoid oils with a particularly high omega-6 to omega-3 ratio:

- Soy: 7:1
- Corn oil: 60:1
- Peanut oil: 32:1
- Safflower oil: 75:1

And these aren't the only fats you should avoid . . .

D. Completely Avoid Trans Fats

Trans fats are bad news, really bad news. Trans fats are a result of food science experimentation and have been conclusively linked to many health problems and diseases. Trans fats are created in the process of saturating an unsaturated liquid fat like vegetable oil with hydrogen (also called hydrogenation) into a solid fat such as margarine. Why would food companies want to solidify unsaturated oils? Because purchasing these cheap vegetable oils and solidifying them through hydrogenation is still much cheaper than using naturally saturated fats (like butter) and also increases shelf life.

Why avoid trans fats? Consider some of these findings:

- The consumption of trans fats is strongly correlated to coronary heart disease.[74]
- The daily intake of about five grams of trans fat is associated with a 25 percent increase in the risk of ischemic heart disease.[75]
- Metabolic studies have shown that trans fats have adverse effects on blood lipid levels—increasing LDL ("bad") cholesterol while decreasing HDL ("good") cholesterol.[76]

The American Heart Foundation recommends severe limitation of trans fats to less than 1 percent of daily calories (roughly two grams), which I think is still too much, as even very small amounts can significantly increase the risk of heart disease. Small amounts of trans fat occur naturally in meat and dairy products, which means that if you consume them, then you should definitely steer clear of all processed foods that contain added trans fats. I recommend zero trans fats; there is no safe amount; even the smallest amounts are harmful.

The bad news continues. According to labeling regulations, if a food contains less than half a gram of trans fat in a serving size, it can be labeled as "No Trans Fats" or "0% Trans Fats." More than four servings of these "trans-fat-free" foods, and you're already over your limit, which is easy to do when a small bag of chips has anywhere from two to four servings. That's why it's especially important to take time to read the label and doublecheck how much trans fat a food contains, rather than trust any health claim on the front of the package. Read the ingredient list, and if it says "trans fats," then don't think twice, just put it back. Because the negative health effects of trans fats has rightly received its fair share of bad press in recent years, and food companies are loath to let go of a cheap source of fat, trans fats are being disguised as "fully hydrogenated" or "partially hydrogenated" oils, or as "shortening." As soon as you see the word "hydrogenated," or any word that even resembles it, you can expect trans fats. Monoglycerides and diglycerides, which are synthetically manufactured and used as emulsifiers in foods, also contain trans fats, and these ingredients also don't need to be labeled as containing these harmful fats.

There is a long list of trans-fat-heavy foods to avoid:

- **Any food deep-fried in fat.** Unless a food is deep fried in a natural saturated fat like lard, which is too expensive for food manufacturers, then it is fried in cheap vegetable oils, and it will contain high amounts of trans fats. Chips, fries, and donuts are all loaded with trans fats. According to one study, the cooking oil used for French fries in McDonald's outlets in the United States contained 23 percent trans fatty acids, with one serving of fries (171 grams) containing ten grams of trans fats.[77]
- **Margarine or vegetable shortening.** Again, come back to real food. I personally don't eat butter, but if I did, I would choose good quality butter over its imitational equivalent margarine, which is usually made from soy and loaded with trans fat.
- **Vegetable oils.** Veggie oils sold commercially in supermarkets are partially hydrogenated to make them more stable; all the more reason to buy good quality oils, if you buy oils at all.

Other foods labels you should be checking (if you decide to eat them):

- Baked goods
- Packaged snack foods
- Breads
- Salad dressings
- Cookies
- Crackers
- Breakfast cereals
- Microwave popcorn (be extra cautious with popcorn, which can be particularly high in trans fats)

- Peanut butter (most commercial peanut butters are loaded with trans fats)
- Sauces
- Frozen pizza
- Breaded fish sticks
- Puddings
- Ramen noodles

Restaurants also use vegetable oils to deep-fry many of their foods. Be sure to ask your server what oil they use if they are deep-frying, or if they are using real butter in their cooking. Eating out in restaurants should generally be avoided, or at least saved for very special occasions.

E. Remember That Calories from Fat Add Up Fast

If weight loss is a part of your goal, then you should consider cutting back on fat. As mentioned, fats are twice as high in calories than proteins and carbohydrates. There are approximately 120 calories in every single tablespoon of extra oil you add to your diet. Butter also packs a mean punch at 100 calories per tablespoon. This adds up fast. You only need to eat about an ounce of nuts or seeds, a couple of tablespoons of flax or chia seeds, or about a half an avocado to satisfy your daily fat requirements.

Most people are simply unaware of how much fat they are eating. Although I generally don't recommend calorie counting, using a calorie counting website like CRON-O-meter for a couple of days to get a better idea of the fat content of foods can be very insightful. When I first did this, even after years of studying nutrition, I was amazed. This is a simple way to bring awareness to the fat content of your most frequently eaten foods. Remember that all fruits and vegetables contain some fat, so you're already getting more fat than you realize just by sticking to fruits and vegetables. Adding a small portion of healthy fats such as avocado, nuts, and seeds to your diet will ensure that you also get your daily dose of essential fatty acids.

6. Work Towards Eliminating Salt Intake

Dietary sodium is essential, but only in small quantities. The average person is consuming anywhere from ten to fifteen times the amount they need. Most people have been hooked on salty foods for so long they consider their salt intake to be normal. The good news is that you can undo this preference for salt by simply giving it up. Similar to how smoking damages taste buds and the ability to taste food, salt also damages the taste buds making food taste bland. The longer you go without salt, the more your taste buds will become sensitive to it, and the more you will notice the rich and delicious flavors of foods. What you now taste as normal will taste very salty to you after a few weeks of not consuming salt.

According to the Center for Disease Control (CDC), approximately 77 percent of sodium comes from packaged, processed, store-bought, restaurant, and fast foods. Only 6 percent of sodium is added at the table and 5 percent during cooking. That makes a total of 88 percent. Eliminating packaged, processed foods is definitely the best and first place to start. Wonder where the other 12 percent of sodium comes from? The last 12 percent is found naturally in whole foods, providing us with all the sodium we need to be healthy.

What Is Our Best Source of Sodium and Potassium?

If you eat a diverse plant-based diet comprised mainly of fresh, organic fruits and vegetables, and you cut out all added salt from your diet, you're not cutting out all sodium—that would be impossible. If you eat a varied plant-based diet, then it will be very difficult for you to eat too little sodium, because sodium is naturally found in most of the whole foods we eat, to varying degrees. Not surprisingly, the proportion of potassium to sodium found in fruits and vegetables mimics the same ratio inside our own cells. I aim for no more than approximately 300–500 mg on the high end of sodium per day and feel like this is an optimal ratio, considering that I'm very active. As soon as I feel like I'm taking in more sodium than my body needs, my body communicates this to me—especially through swelling of my fingers, dry mouth, and excess water retention.

Here are some great sources of plant foods that contain healthy amounts of sodium (source: USDA Nutrient Database):

- Coconut water, 1 cup, 252 mg
- Honeydew melon, 1 medium, 205 mg
- Swiss chard, 2 cups, 154 mg
- Cantaloupe melon, 1 medium, 88 mg
- Carrots, 2 medium, 84 mg
- Sweet potato, 1 medium, 72 mg
- Beet, 1 medium (2 inches), 64 mg
- Celery, 2 stalks, 64 mg
- Kale, 2 cups, 58 mg
- Spinach, 2 cups, 48 mg

My goal is not to vilify sodium—sodium is essential; we just don't need it in the form of salt and we don't need as much of it as most people are consuming. As the Institute of Medicine so poignantly stated in the conclusion of a report titled *Strategies to Reduce Sodium Intake in the United States*: "In the face of chronic disease risks associated with sodium intake, the current level of sodium in the food supply—added by food manufacturers, food-service operators, and restaurants—is too high to be 'safe.'"[78] I think that pretty much sums it up.

Considering that approximately 40 percent of our collective food dollars are spent eating out, it is very difficult to know how much sodium we are truly consuming. Again, you limit your intake just by skipping the restaurant all together and instead preparing your own delicious foods at home. That being said, just because you prepare foods at home (unless you're only consuming whole foods), it doesn't mean that you're skipping the salt. Many packaged foods that we use to prepare meals are also high in salt. The more you increase your intake of fruits and vegetables, the less you will have to worry about how much sodium you're consuming.

Low-Sodium Grocery Shopping

As you are transitioning, it's essential that you learn how to navigate the grocery store and read food labels so you can make informed decisions. When it comes to grocery shopping for you and your family, it's important to be aware of how ubiquitous salt is. Salt is used in many kinds of food-processing techniques. When buying foods at the grocery store (and while eating out), beware of these top ten food-preparation methods that are sure to be high in sodium.

1. Canned
2. Pickled
3. Corned
4. Breaded
5. Barbecued
6. Brined
7. Smoked
8. Seasoned
9. Au gratin
10. Cured

Sodium and Food Labeling

The Food and Drug Administration has guidelines that outline the terms a company can use when describing sodium content on the label of prepared foods. I highly recommend transitioning towards limiting and cutting out packaged and processed foods from your diet. If you choose to buy any packaged foods, take the time to read the label and avoid foods that contain more than 35 mg of sodium in a serving. Also be aware of serving size. One of the ways that food companies can trick consumers about sodium content is to make the serving size smaller than what you would normally consume in one sitting.

Sodium free	Less than 5 mg of sodium per portion
Very low sodium	Less than 35 mg of sodium per portion
Low sodium	Less than 140 mg of sodium per portion
Reduced sodium	Contains 25 percent less sodium than original food item
Light in sodium	Contains 50 percent less than original food item
Unsalted/No added salt/Without salt added	Absolutely no salt has been added to a food that's normally processed with salt

When reading the ingredients list, be aware that sodium can also be called or listed as:

1. Salt (sodium chloride)
2. Sodium sulfite
3. Sodium alginate
4. Sodium caseinate
5. Disodium phosphate
6. Sodium benzoate
7. Sodium hydroxide
8. Sodium citrate
9. Sodium propionate

10. Baking powder
11. Baking soda
12. Sodium bicarbonate
13. Monosodium glutamate (MSG)

Some people find it easier to wean themselves off salt slowly. A great way to kick the salt habit is to transition to seaweeds like dulse or kelp. Seaweeds also have quite a bit of salt, so it's a good idea to rinse them before you eat them to reduce the sodium content, and use sparingly. When making food at home, instead of adding salt, use fresh herbs like cilantro, parsley, dill, basil, and oregano to add flavor to your meals. You can also try dried seasoning herbs or use fresh lemon to add a naturally zesty flavor to a meal.

7. Choose Your Grains Wisely, If You Must Eat Them at All

Many health professionals advocate that grains are a part of a healthy diet. Due to the decades of government marketing of "the four food groups" and the food pyramid, it's become taboo to say that grains are not, in fact, a health food. Of course, replacing meat, dairy products, and refined grains with *whole* grains and legumes is a step in the right direction, as many studies have shown, but this doesn't make them an *ideal* food source. Eating grains every day has become the norm, but just because everyone else is doing it doesn't make it a good idea! Grains are nutritionally inferior to fruits and vegetables and definitely don't taste as good (unless loaded with refined sugar, fat, and salt).

"Just as the tobacco industry created and sustained its market with the addictive properties of cigarettes, so does wheat in the diet make for a helpless, hungry consumer. From the perspective of the seller of food products, wheat is a perfect processed food ingredient: The more you eat, the more you want. The situation for the food industry has been made even better by the glowing endorsements provided by the US government urging Americans to eat more 'healthy' whole grains."

—William Davis, *Wheat Belly*

Think of it from an intuitive perspective. If you were to walk up to a field of wheat or an orchard of cherry trees filled with plump red cherries, which would you naturally gravitate toward? Which one just made your mouth water? We need machines and technology to be able to consume wheat as a reliable fuel source. Fruits and vegetables are our best sources of vitamins and minerals, and grains are low in many of these essential nutrients. Grains are also high in *anti*-nutrients like phytic acid, tannins, enzyme inhibitors, and lectins that inhibit the body from absorbing nutrients from these foods.

Grains, like meat and dairy, are also acidic to the body. The body needs to maintain a narrow blood pH range of about 7.4, slightly alkaline. Think of alkalinity as the opposing force to acidity. When we eat grains (or meat or dairy) that are high in acidic minerals, our bodies need to neutralize the acidity entering our blood with an alkaline base in order to maintain homeostasis or balance. The body then responds by leaching calcium (an alkaline mineral) from our bones, which weakens our bones and makes us susceptible to bone loss and fractures. If you take your health seriously, at least 80 percent of your diet should consist of alkaline foods. Guess what foods are alkaline to the body? Let me hear you say it with me: *Fruits and vegetables!*

Hooked on Wheat

Many people eat wheat at every single meal without even knowing it. What's worse is that many people are actually addicted to wheat—also without knowing it. Wheat is an insidious grain, hidden in many prepared, packaged, and store-bought food, including breads, bagels, pasta, cereals, cakes, cookies, and even beer. Wheat flour is also added to many products, including soy sauce, ketchup, processed meats, and even ice cream!

When I think of wheat, I think of *cravings*. Wheat will always make you want to keep going back for more, and it is often the reason for many people's food obsession, the culprit (along with other grain-based, hyper-palatable food products) that keeps you hooked on your struggle with food. Wheat is a very common addictive food, because, like cheese, dairy products, and hyper-palatable foods, wheat also contains opioids, producing the familiar hyper-pleasurable response, similar to morphine and other drugs.

If weight loss is one of your health goals, I would strongly encourage you to remove all wheat and wheat-related products from your diet. Wheat is not only an appetite stimulant; it also sends your blood sugar levels on a roller coaster ride—except this ride isn't any fun, and for the sake of your health, you might want to step off. What you want are stable blood sugar levels, the kind of stability you get from eating a diet that consists mostly of fresh fruits and vegetables.

Gliadins and glutenins, the two main components of gluten found in wheat, cause an inflammatory response in the body—also not good for your health. Chronic low-level inflammation has been linked to many diseases, ranging from diabetes,[79] arthritis, heart disease,[80] autoimmune diseases,[81] depression, osteoporosis, and aging of the skin, not to mention overweight and obesity. Wheat is also one of the top seven food allergens, containing more than eighty different components that can cause a negative reaction.[82]

What You Need to Know About Gluten

Gluten is a protein found in grains like wheat, rye, spelt, and barley. The term "gluten free" (GF) has increasingly become a mainstream nutritional catchphrase, and for good reason. It is estimated that about 10-15 percent of the population is gluten intolerant, with some estimates going as high as 50 percent.[83] Many diseases and hundreds of symptoms have been related to gluten intolerance. Even if you've never been officially diagnosed, you may still be dealing with some level of sensitivity to gluten, as the vast majority of gluten-intolerant individuals are never diagnosed.

Full-blown celiac disease (allergy to gluten) causes an autoimmune-type reaction in the body in which the body reacts so strongly it damages the delicate lining of the small intestine, causing chronic malabsorption of nutrients.[84] For sensitive individuals, gluten causes body-wide inflammation triggering insulin resistance, which causes weight gain and diabetes, as well as over 55 conditions including autoimmune diseases, irritable bowel, reflux, cancer, depression, osteoporosis, and more.[85]

The worst part is that many people who are allergic to wheat and gluten don't know they are intolerant, nor do they know that this intolerance actually ends up causing cravings to these foods, creating a very unpleasant cycle also known as *hooked*. If you frequently binge on wheat products and feel like it's incredibly difficult to go even a day without wheat, this is a telltale sign you have wheat or gluten intolerance.

" . . . a third to half of all people who have these reactions actually end up craving the very food that is causing them health problems. Wheat in particular is a common food allergen, addictant, and trigger to cravings, and there are real physiological reasons why this occurs . . . "

—**Melissa Smith**, *Going Against the Grain*

Off the Wheat Hook

If you feel your relationship with food is like being caught in a vise grip, try giving up all wheat from your diet for thirty days, and see how you feel after the trial period. Just like we wouldn't advise a cocaine addict to "cut back a little," it will be easier on you if you go "cold turkey" on this one. Don't just cut back, go all the way, and make sure you read labels if you continue to buy anything that comes in a package. Withdrawal symptoms are common to substance dependence and withdrawal from wheat is no joke (a good indication of how addictive it is). You may experience symptoms during this time of wheat abstinence, including cravings, nausea, anxiety, and headaches.

Sure, labels that read "gluten free" are better than eating gluten, but don't get caught in the marketing hype; gluten-free pizza and cookies are still pizza and cookies! Just because it's gluten-free doesn't mean it's healthy; these are still highly processed foods, usually full of sugar, fat, and salt.

I'm not telling you to *never* eat any grains or starches ever again. Like all the recommendations outlined in this chapter, it's for you to decide and draw your own conclusion. Since they are nutritionally inferior to fruits and vegetables, I recommend experimenting with removing them from your diet and see how you feel. Go at whatever pace feels good for you. If you eat grains every day, try cutting down to once a week, or once a month. I very rarely eat any grains, and I don't miss them one bit. I immediately notice how bland they taste and gassy and bloated they make me feel, so what's to miss?

If you would like to continue eating grains, choose them wisely. Try eating only whole grains that you cook at home and avoid all packed and processed foods that contain refined grains (even if the label states "Contains Whole Grains" on the package.) It's also a good idea to steer clear of wheat all together and choose gluten-free grains instead. These include:

- Quinoa
- Buckwheat (Buckwheat is technically not a grain, which makes this option even better. Buckwheat flour makes for a great wheat-flour alternative. On occasion, I like to make raw, sprouted buckwheat granola for breakfast. Check out www.happyandraw.com for a simple buckwheat granola recipe.)
- Amaranth
- Millet
- Wild rice

If you do decide to eat grains, avoid slathering them with high-sugar, high-fat, high-salt "additions." Instead try adding a healthier grain choice like quinoa into a homemade vegetable soup or stew, or sprinkle a little bit of whole grain on top of a salad.

Pause & Reflect: Letting Go of What No Longer Serves You

I know it can be challenging to question your eating habits. Allow yourself to feel whatever you need to feel about the information presented in this chapter: angry and upset that many of the foods you eat many not be the best choices, or maybe happy to finally feel validated and supported to move in a new direction. Take a moment to reflect on the following questions:

1. What processed foods that you incorporate into your life are you now ready to let go of?

2. Are you willing to see that most foods that stock the supermarket shelves are heavily refined, processed, and perhaps not "normal" to consume?

3. Are you ready to accept that dieting is not a long-term sustainable solution to weight loss and that what is required is an integrated lifestyle approach?

Off the Hook

You can help end your food and weight struggle for good by adopting and working towards a lower-fat, lower-salt diet, primarily consisting of real, whole foods in the form of fresh, organic fruits and vegetables. It's easier than you think, and it's an incredibly tasty way to live. By following the simple guidelines in this chapter, you will immediately start to notice positive changes in your body, your mind, and in your spirit.

Perhaps you're one of those people, like many of my clients, who know *what* to do but have a hard time actually doing it. It takes more than simply knowing the information regarding what to eat. When it comes to our relationship with food, there's much to take into consideration. You may already be rooted in behavioral patterns that are at odds with the seven dietary guidelines discussed in this chapter. Again, this links back to *how*—how to make the changes when you may already be entrenched in behavioral patterns that don't support a healthy lifestyle. The next step is to look at your behavioral patterns and create a roadmap to help you implement the healthy dietary changes that you are seeking to make.

PART THREE

The Behavioral Hook

"Your beliefs become your thoughts,
Your thoughts become your words,
Your words become your actions,
Your actions become your habits,
Your habits become your values,
Your values become your destiny."
—Mahatma Gandhi

Chapter 5

How Our
Behavioral Patterns Hook Us

You might be familiar with this scenario. You set a New Year's resolution: This year is going to be different. This year you're going to change. You're going to kick that unhealthy habit that no longer serves you, get into the best shape of your life, and shed those excess pounds you've been carrying. The *thought* of change feels good, doesn't it? But what about actually *implementing* those changes?

How about this scenario: It's Sunday night. You promise yourself that this time you're going to make it happen: tomorrow you're going on a diet (aka restriction). You had the "perfect" day on Monday. Tuesday night is movie night. You walk into the theater, and wham, the smell of popcorn filling the lobby overwhelms you, and then you see it in plain sight. You're hooked. Without thinking, you walk over, and before you know it you have an extra-large bucket of popcorn in your hands. Caught off guard by the first little road bump, in that instant you give up all hope. Two months and ten pounds later, you're ready to make another promise to yourself: this time you're going to change.

If you are familiar with this all-or-nothing mentality, you may be wondering how you can create a path for yourself that is a little more sane, a little more balanced, and a little more in the direction of achieving your goals. Maybe you've heard all this information about the benefits of fruits and vegetables and the health risks of chronic consumption of refined sugar, fat, and salt before. Maybe you've even agreed with every single word I've written and want nothing more than to jump into these lifestyle changes, but you feel unable to override old habits and adopt these new behaviors.

Meet my client, Michelle. Like many other people I've worked with, Michelle knows what she wants but finds it challenging to stick to the changes she longs to implement. Everyone struggles to some degree with kicking old habits. We all know it can be extremely frustrating, not to mention discouraging, when we do something we promised ourselves (for the thousandth time) that we weren't going to do. This is simply part of what it means to be human.

Why does it feel so hard and so overwhelming to actually follow through on change? You know you want to lose weight, for example, yet the temptation of the pizza, the fried foods—insert your own food temptation here—keeps catching you off guard. Sometimes you may not even realize that you've succumbed yet again until after you've given in. Did some entity just temporarily take over your mind while you acted unconsciously, on automatic pilot? What's going on here?

One Brain—Two Worlds Apart

From a neuroscience perspective, the brain has two very separate and distinct, not to mention contrasting and conflicting, minds.[86] I'm sure you know what I'm talking about. You've been eating well all week, and then all of a sudden you're triggered—there it is, the box of cookies. You go back and forth with the ping-pong match in your head . . .

"I want it . . . "

"But you shouldn't have it . . . "

"But I've been doing so well all week . . . "

"But you'll regret it later; you know you will feel horrible . . . "

"But what about just one?"

"You know you can't eat just one . . . you've never been able to eat just one!"

Interesting how we can even phrase it as "I" and "you," as if we are two separate people in that moment talking to each other. Although we have one brain, we actually have two separate minds.*

---

* The first time I heard this concept was on Kelly McGonigal's audio course *The Neuroscience of Change* by Sounds True. Please refer to this excellent resource for more information on this topic.

1. **Automatic (or unconscious) mind.** This part of our mind is rooted in controlling habitual patterns of response and often drives unconscious behaviors. It acts on impulse and is triggered by stress and other instinctual survival-based mechanisms. This mind is what pushes us to forgo our values and long-term goals and seek out immediate gratification. The majority of the thousands of decisions we make on a daily basis are made unconsciously with this automatic mind.

2. **Conscious mind.** This is the part of our mind that can delay instant gratification and immediate pleasure for the achievement of longer-term goals. I introduced you to your powerful prefrontal cortex (PFC) in chapter 3, the most evolved part of your brain that supports willed action and self-control, and helps you to resist temptation. Your conscious mind is intimately connected to this part of your brain. It creates the awareness that you may not want to eat that pizza because it doesn't align with your long-term vision of health and well-being. This mind allows you to remember what you want—is it really that pizza, or rather to fit into your slim jeans? This mind is more rational, intentional, wise, and self-aware.

Each "mind" is linked to separate neural circuits in the brain. The area of the brain responsible for creating and maintaining habits, the automatic mind, also shares very close neural circuitry with the areas of the brain responsible for survival, like sexual desire, stress, and the fear response, as well as hunger and appetite control. This explains why many people who struggle with changing habits are usually struggling to change unhealthy habits related to one of these survival-based mechanisms. The good news is that practicing simple mindfulness techniques (discussed in chapters 8 and 10) can strengthen your conscious mind and allow you to more easily follow through on your goals.

Defining Habits

Repeating a behavior forms a habit. We can tell something has become a habit when we've done it so often the actions become almost involuntary. It is this "involuntary" tendency that makes habits more difficult to give up. When you feel stressed (trigger) and you reach for food (reward), this develops a neurological pathway in your brain. The more you repeat this behavior, the stronger the pathway in the brain becomes. Think of it this way; every time you repeat a behavior, you're adding a thread from A (trigger) to B (reward) in your brain until eventually it becomes a very thick rope.

The good news is that if you don't act out that habit, over time the rope can weaken and wither away.

Changing what you eat can be challenging, but it is possible and achievable. However, it takes dedication, focus, and commitment. With the right intentions and underlying motivations—and the will to see your highest goals manifest— change is possible.

The Automatic Mind

Your brain is designed to be efficient and conserve energy—another fundamental survival-based capacity. As a result, your brain allows the patterns you repeat regularly to bypass conscious thought as a way of saving time and energy, creating habitual patterns of response. It would be exhausting to have to constantly think about every single decision you make each day. That's why the brain is built to hold onto, remember, and then streamline repeated behaviors. The behaviors that you perform every day, like brushing your teeth, tying your shoelaces, eating, and driving to work tend to become automatic, without you having to consciously think about what you're doing.

Sure, efficiency and streamlining behavior can be great, but what about when it comes to our food choices? You may be like the millions of other people who use food as a coping mechanism— perhaps for emotional support, to comfort yourself, to calm yourself down, or as your primary source of pleasure in life. Repeating these eating patterns year after year reinforces them, even to the point where these food patterns and the purpose they serve for you are now outside of your conscious awareness.

You may be thinking: "If I've been creating these habits for so many years, how am I ever going to change?" Fortunately, you can take this information and use it to your advantage. You can choose to step out of automatic mode and into conscious awareness mode. The brain is really good at learning *new* habits, and as we will see, the best way to give up old unhealthy habits is to replace them with new healthier ones. Then these new patterns can cruise on automatic pilot (with a healthy degree of continued self-awareness) to support you in your journey to health.

Stress and the Automatic Mind

As discussed in chapter 1, we can get cued by any number of things, and this cue can trigger a habitual response. It can be a place, a thought, an emotion, a person, the sight of your dinner plate—anything can cause an unconscious reaction. One of the strongest cues that trigger us happens to be something that runs rampant in our culture: stress.

Stress pushes us from our conscious mind to our automatic mind because our stress response was initially rooted in survival, sharing a similar neural circuitry in the brain. The nature of stress has drastically changed, and today we're experiencing high amounts of stress that aren't rooted in life-or-death situations but rather are more often based on *perceptions* of stress, whether it be social, work, financial, health, or family related.

Kelly McGonigal, author of *The Willpower Instinct: How Self Control Works, Why It Matters, and What You Can Do To Get More of It* (a book I highly recommend), states:

Each of these "minds" are supported by different neural circuits—different systems of the brain in command of your thoughts, emotions, and actions. Stress selectively inhibits the circuitry of self-awareness and self-control, and activates the circuitry of habit and impulse. Neuroscientists describe it like flicking a switch: stress hormones turn off the reflection mode and turn on the reflex mode.[87]

Basically, stress inhibits our ability to adapt and implement the changes we want to make. Research shows that you can actually push people toward habitual behaviors at the expense of their goals by stressing them out.[88] Stress impairs the functioning of the prefrontal cortex, which we rely on to help us make decisions that are in our best (long-term) interest, and which actually improves the performance of simpler, well-rehearsed tasks[89] (aka habits). Stress also impairs higher-order prefrontal cortex abilities such as working memory and attention regulation. And that's not all. According to Dr. Sara Gottfried, author of *The Hormone Cure*: " . . . prolonged exposure to high cortisol constricts blood flow to the brain. That adversely affects brain function, decreases your emotional intelligence, and accelerates age-related cognitive function."[90]

The impact of stress on our body and overall health can be devastating. Stress is not only associated with impaired mental functioning and an obstacle when it comes to creating new healthier habits, but it is increasingly being associated with a wide range of diseases. Gottfried also states that "Stress is the top reason behind most visits to the doctor, and it contributes to all the big causes of death, including heart disease, diabetes, stroke, and cancer."[91] According to *New York Times* bestselling author and family physician Dr. Mark Hyman, "Ninety-five percent of disease is either caused by or worsened by stress."[92] This makes stress management a top health priority.

Learning to manage and cope with stress in healthy ways is essential for you on this journey. What do you normally turn to for support when you're feeling the weight of stress in your life? In 2011, the American Psychological Association found that approximately 34 percent of people who feel stressed tend to overeat and turn to unhealthy foods, 27 percent say they skip meals, and about 42 percent say they lie awake at night.[93] My primary recommendation for managing stress is meditation (discussed in chapter 10), but there are many other things that you can do to immediately start feeling more calm, relaxed, and at ease in your body and in your life. Spending time with loved ones, spending time in nature, connecting with the earth, spending time in your garden, laughing, singing, playing games, listening to music, dancing, low-intensity exercise, baths, massage, acupuncture, calling a friend, relaxation techniques, visualization, spending time with pets, curling up with a good book—all these activities not only help you feel good, but simultaneously help reduce stress. It's just a matter of making time for them and incorporating these activities in your life. An additional bonus is that healthy stress management helps release and relieve any dependency on habitual eating choices that have served as a coping mechanism to help get you through stressful times.

There is another type of stress that also inhibits our chances of transitioning to a new and healthier lifestyle: self-criticism.

A Motivating Force: Self-Compassion Versus Self-Criticism

Motivation: It's what we all want, yet find difficult to get—or at least hold on to. We have this misconception that we need to be very strict with ourselves, playing the role of self-disciplinarian to reach our health goals, whether the goal is weight loss or change of dietary habits. We've been taught that self-discipline is a superior strategy than self-compassion for following through on commitments. We've confused *self-discipline* (most often paired with self-criticism) with *motivation* and believe that if we are not impersonating a drill sergeant, reprimanding ourselves, and following every single dietary rule to a T, we're sure to fail. We believe that being hard on ourselves by making ourselves feel bad about what we just did (or didn't do) will motivate us to change. What an unfortunate delusion we've created!

Self-criticism is a form of negative self-judgment and self-evaluation that can be directed to various aspects of the self, such as one's physical appearance, behavior, inner thoughts and emotions, personality, and intellectual attributes.[94]

Ready for some great news? Being self-critical doesn't motivate us but in fact drains us of the energy we might have otherwise had to reach our goals in the first place! Research overwhelmingly points counter to all previous logic: the harder you are on yourself, the less likely you are to succeed. Self-compassion creates more motivation than self-criticism, and more motivation means a greater chance of success. Self-compassion fosters the inner strength and initiative we need to follow through on our goals or make changes that we've found hard to maintain in the past. Research now shows that self-compassionate people are less likely to give up on and lose sight of their goals and exhibit more self-control and self-initiative than their self-critical counterparts.[95] Other research findings from Abant Izzet Baysal University demonstrated that self-kindness, awareness of common humanity, and mindfulness (the three components of compassion, as we'll see below) related positively to motivation, while self-judgment and isolation related negatively to motivation.[96]

Essentially, by being self-critical you're setting yourself up for failure; it's like chaining a dead weight to your motivation while trying to summon the strength to make the dietary or lifestyle changes you've thus far been unable to make. Being self-critical activates the neural networks in your brain responsible for self-punishment and behavioral inhibition.[97] Self-criticism basically stops you dead in your tracks, and prevents you from getting to where you ultimately want to go.

Not only does self-compassion translate into more motivation than self-criticism, this characteristic just so happens to also have many other life-enhancing benefits. People who score higher in self-compassion tend to have lower levels of depression, anxiety, and eating disorders, are happier and more optimistic, and experience greater social connection.[98] Self-criticism, on the other hand, is inversely correlated to these behavioral outcomes.[99] In one study, Dr. Kristin Neff, a pioneer in the field of self-compassion and professor at the University of Texas, tracked participants for an entire month to observe the difference self-compassion can make. She found that practicing self-compassion had the same effect as antidepressants *but without the side effects.* It improved their positive emotional state and at the same time weakened their negative mental state for the duration of the month.[100] Consider Neff's perspective: "Self-compassion is really conducive to motivation. The reason you don't let your children eat five big tubs of ice cream is because you care about them. With self-compassion, if you care about yourself, you do what's healthy for you rather than what's harmful to you."

What Is Self-Compassion?

Compassion can be defined as a deep awareness of the suffering of another coupled with the wish to relieve it. With this same definition in mind, we can view self-compassion as the awareness of our own suffering with the same wish to relieve it. Just as we would like to relieve the pain of others, we can also develop a heartfelt wish to relieve ourselves of the same pain. When you are feeling sad, upset, angry, lonely, frustrated, stressed, or—insert emotion here—self-compassion is the act of being gentle, patient, loving, and supportive with yourself.

"Self-compassion is the missing ingredient in every diet and weight-loss strategy."

—**Jean Fain,** *The Self-Compassion Diet*

The Three Components of Compassion

According to Neff, self-compassion is comprised of three essential elements: mindfulness, self-kindness, and common humanity.[101]

1. *Mindfulness* is the capacity to be present for and look at whatever emotions arise without judgment. We will discuss mindfulness in chapter 7 and also look at how to work with emotions from this mindful perspective in chapter 10.
2. *Self-kindness* points to the ways we can be warm and understanding toward ourselves instead of dishing out harsh criticisms when we slip up, fail, or fall off the proverbial wagon. When we are kind and soften our hearts toward ourselves, we learn to be gentler, more accepting, and loving.
3. *Shared humanity* is a mindset of "us" rather than "me." By practicing compassion, we dissolve the separateness and connect to our common humanity—that we all experience hardship and suffering and that this is part of what it means to be human. In this way we can reach out, even if in

our own minds and hearts, and know that we are not alone. This is how we foster compassion for others and ourselves.

"Only when we know our own darkness well can we be present with the darkness of others. Compassion becomes real when we recognize our shared humanity."

—**Pema Chödrön,** *The Places That Scare You*

Self-Compassion Versus Self-Accountability

Many people think that after they slip up they need to hold themselves accountable for their mistakes by getting angry, upset, or down on themselves. We may have learned this approach from childhood as our parents reprimanded us when we did something wrong. In children, the self-control center in the brain is still developing, and so they need guidance from parents to learn what's acceptable or not. Sometimes the message doesn't get across as lovingly as it should, and so as adults we take on that role of the overbearing parents in our own minds. But self-criticism is not the way to hold ourselves accountable; self-compassion is.

Self-compassion actually increases personal responsibility for an undesirable event by recognizing mistakes, thereby increasing the likelihood of self-regulation in the future.[102] According to Kelly McGonigal, "It's forgiveness, not guilt, that increases accountability. Researchers have found that seeing personal failure through a self-compassionate point of view makes people more likely to take personal responsibility for the failure than when they take a self-critical point of view . . . and [they are] more likely to learn from the experience."[103]

Self-accountability doesn't have to include any degree of criticism whatsoever—and it's actually better for you if it doesn't. Accountability just allows you to shine the light of awareness on your behavior and decide whether this behavior is serving or hurting you. If you can look at it and honestly know that it's not serving you but in fact hurting you quite deeply, you can let this awareness guide your decisions in the future.

If you have already spiraled out of control, after a binge perhaps, allow yourself the space to see clearly what you've done without self-condemnation or self-criticism. This keeps you from digging a deeper hole. Self-compassion involves recognizing mistakes without becoming overwhelmed with negative emotions, thereby increasing your chances of making better choices that are more aligned with your values and future goals.[104]

Self-Compassion: A Ticket for Self-Indulgence?

In her research, Neff found that "the biggest reason people aren't more self-compassionate is that they are afraid they'll become self-indulgent. They believe self-criticism is what keeps them in line. Most people have gotten it wrong because our culture says being hard on yourself is the way to be."[105] Self-compassion does not, by any means, equal self-indulgence. When you practice self-compassion, it's not about giving yourself the green light to eat every last donut within a ten-mile radius. It doesn't mean giving yourself an excuse to overindulge, or to ignore the fact that you're upset. Self-compassion is not about denial; it's about *acceptance*. Researchers Adams and Leary from Wake Forest University found that even a minor dose of self-compassion instruction prevented future self-indulgence, especially among restrictive and guilty eaters.[106] Two separate groups of women were instructed to eat a donut. One group received informal words of self-compassion ("everyone eats unhealthy sometimes, so I don't think there's any reason to feel bad about it"), while the other group did not. The group that received the compassionate guidance ate less of the subsequent bowl of candies that the researchers put out than the group of women who didn't receive any self-compassionate advice.

"A spoonful of self-compassion makes it possible to have a bowl of ice cream without polishing off the whole pint."

—Jean Fain, *The Self-Compassion Diet*

When you practice self-compassion, what you're doing is removing that unnecessary dead weight that is inhibiting you from getting where you want to go. Just this act alone helps you to drop many additional layers of the self-imposed struggle. You are then freer to develop new habits that serve your highest goals by becoming more discriminating about what you want to put in your body from a place of love, respect, and compassion for yourself. You can get to a point where you experience a trigger or food craving and say, "I don't need that; I don't even want it," without an ounce of struggle. You can develop a sincere desire to end your suffering by ending your dependence on things that cause that suffering by developing new habits rooted in self-compassion.

Getting Unhooked

Although the brain is geared towards habitual patterns, it is also very good at learning new patterns and behaviors—as long as you flex your conscious mind. One of the ways we strengthen our conscious mind and make healthier habits in spite of the default of the automatic mind is to practice mindfulness, which we will discuss in Part 4. The other way that we strengthen our conscious minds is to create a clear vision of what you ultimately want to achieve. We will explore this visionary process in the next chapter, which includes identifying your underlying purpose and motivation, and then setting goals to achieve your vision, wrapping the whole process in an attitude of self-compassion and kindness.

Chapter 6

Unhooked: Committing to Change

You may have promised yourself big changes in the past and are now skeptical of your ability to fully commit and follow through. Let that go; it's now in the past. Holding on to or focusing on your past mistakes will only make it harder for you to move forward. Bring yourself to the present moment and look at how ready you are for change in this moment, right here and now.

Allow me to introduce you to a very important concept that will bolster your confidence in your ability to change: the power of *neuroplasticity*. This term refers to your brain's ability to change, to literally re-wire by creating new neural pathways due to changes in behavior. It doesn't matter how old you are; your brain has the ability to adapt to a new way of living. Every time you engage in a new behavior or think new thoughts, neural pathways are forged, and with repetition new habits are strengthened.

Ending your struggle with food will require you to learn new habits that will forge new pathways in your brain. One way you encourage brain plasticity is through a mindful, goal-directed approach. Grab your journal; you're going to need it!

Painting the Big-Picture Perspective

Okay, it's time to dive in. Research shows that there are a number of ways you can increase your chances of successful change. One technique involves adopting a "big picture" perspective of your life. I invite you to "step out of your life" for just a moment; simply step back and look at your life as an outside observer. It's as if you're looking at actors on the screen, and one of those actors is you! In a perfect world, in terms of your health, what do you see? What is the big-picture perspective of your health-related goals? What does it look like, *feel like*, to be there? What is your deepest desire and underlying motivation in achieving this goal?

Now step back into your life and look at where you currently are. You're going from a broad perspective to a narrow focus. Do you see a difference between where you are now and where you want to be? What do you have to do *specifically* (how, when, and where) to get there? What are you willing to commit to in order to achieve the bigger picture of what you actually *want*?

This technique helps strengthen your prefrontal cortex (PFC), helps reduce impulsivity, and strengthens your ability to consciously choose rather than reach for something out of a habitual, "knee jerk" reaction. This approach provides guidance and structure and will facilitate the creation of new habits. It will also encourage you to follow through on your commitments and support you in reaching your goals.

Defining Vision, Purpose, and Goals

The following process is rooted in this big-picture perspective. Start by creating a personal health *vision statement*. Next, look at the deeper meaning, your underlying motivations, and values that support this vision through a *purpose statement*. Then define and *set goals* to achieve your vision, followed up by an *action plan* to reach each individual goal. This process allows you to focus on your existing values and whether you are living in alignment with them. If one of your highest values is to be healthy and you find yourself making less than healthy choices, you know that you are compromising your highest values and ultimately what you'd like to see manifest as the vision for your future.

Write a Vision Statement

Your personal health vision statement represents *what* you desire to see manifest as a result of your efforts. In Stephen Covey's bestselling book *The Seven Habits of Highly Effective People*, Habit 2 is "begin with the end in mind."[107] This self-discovery step and clarification of highest values and important life goals is the first step to any successful journey: start with the end result in mind.

Your vision statement expresses and paints a vivid mental picture of your ideal future, articulating what the future will be like, *feel* like, and look like when your highest health goals are achieved. This vision can be one year, five years, or even ten years from now. This will allow you to identify the goals you need to set to make this vision a reality.

Exercise # 1: My Personal Health Vision Statement (Begin with the End in Mind)

Take out a pen and paper and get comfortable. Take a moment to imagine yourself sitting exactly where you are, at a specific date in the future. Everything has unfolded exactly the way you envisioned it would. In relation to your health, you are living the life of your dreams. Feel your body. What does it feel like to be in your body? How do you feel physically, mentally, emotionally, and spiritually? Make your vision clear and concise using descriptive language in the present tense. In this process, unleash your imagination and dream big. You may want to use sentences like:

- I feel fit, strong, and healthy.
- I feel well rested.
- I feel energetic and alive.
- I eat delicious whole foods.
- I get lots of exercise; walking every day is something I love to do.
- I'm grateful for my life.

Take as much time as you need to complete your personal health vision statement. This can be an unfolding and developing vision. You don't have to complete it all in one sitting, but you can start jotting down ideas of what your ideal future in your body, mind, and spirit looks like.

Write a Purpose Statement

The purpose statement is the "why"—the heart and soul of why you really want to achieve this beautiful vision. Ultimately, this connects you to your life's deeper meaning and purpose while naturally connecting you to your core values. Think of this process as peeling the layers of an onion. You might start by describing your more superficial motivations, but as you peel away the layers you see what's at the core of your deepest desire for change. Dig deeper and connect to the feeling that reaching these goals will provide for you. When you attach a deeper feeling to why this is important to you, you connect to your highest purpose in life, and you have a better chance of maintaining your goals instead of falling back into old habits during times of stress, distraction, or fatigue.

Exercise #2: My Personal Health Purpose Statement

After you complete your vision statement, you are now ready to write your purpose statement. An effective purpose statement uses powerful words that convey passion and inspires you. It solidifies the motivations behind your purpose. *Why* do you want to reach this vision of health that you've set? Every time you come up with an answer, ask yourself *why* one more time to this new answer, until you can't go any further. Jot down your answers as they come up, and imagine that you are peeling back layers to get to the core of your motivation. An example of this might look something like:

- "I want to lose weight so I can fit into my bikini."
  Dig deeper, what's underneath this motivation? Why do you want to look good in your bikini?
- "Because I want to feel attractive."
  Why? What's underlying this desire to be attractive?
- "I want to feel good in my body."
  Again ask yourself why? What's underlying this?
- "I want freedom from my struggle with food."
- "I truly want to get the most out of life—to experience life fully—and I know I need to be healthy to support that vision."
- "I want to have the energy to play with my kids; they are most important to me."
- "When I am feeling healthy in my body, mind, and spirit, I am a creative channel that allows the most inspiration to flow through my life."

We all have a purpose. We express our purpose and vision with the values we live by and express each day—even if we don't realize it. Make a list of your core values. These might include respect, harmony, independence, health, generosity, compassion, communion with nature, etc. Simply start by brainstorming—jotting down key words, ideas, or phrases—and don't edit or censor yourself at this point; you can always refine your purpose over time.

When writing your purpose statement, connect to what brings you the most joy in life. Explore such thoughts as:

1. I feel my best when . . .
2. What I love to do the most with my time is . . .
3. I feel the most joy in my life when. . .
4. The people I love to help are. . .
5. If money wasn't a consideration, I would spend my time doing . . .

Take as long as you like to write out your purpose statement.

Goal Setting

Now that you've painted a picture of your healthy lifestyle and defined the purpose and value system underlying that vision, it's time to focus on specifics. In this step, you identify and set specific goals that are directly aligned with your larger vision and purpose. Then, outline the action plan you will take to get there. There is a greater chance that you will follow through on your goals when you write them down and stay accountable to someone: a mentor, friend, coach, or loved one. Align with someone you know who can offer you words of loving support. Refer back to chapter 2 for tips on surrounding yourself with a strong social network.

Setting specific goals is about establishing basic guidelines as a road map to help you navigate your way. First, you set your goals, and then you create an action plan, detailing what you need to do to put this plan into action. This plan outlines how, when, where, and possibly even with whom you might be playing out these goal-oriented actions.

Exercise #3: Setting Your Goals

As you start setting goals, try to keep them in the present tense, as this is the reality you wish to manifest. Frame your energy-related goals in a positive rather than negative perspective. For example:

Negative: "I stop eating packaged foods."

Positive: "I eat mostly fruits and vegetables."

Negative: "I force myself to stop eating large portions."

Positive: "I am able to recognize my satiety and to stop eating when I want to."

Your goals should be realistic and feasible, breaking down larger goals into smaller ones so you do not become overwhelmed. As soon as you set unrealistically high goals for yourself, you may be falling into an all-or-nothing mentality, and increasing your risk of failure.

At this point, make a list of your top ten goals, and then circle the top three goals on which you would like to focus.

My Top 10 Goals:

1.

2.

3.

4.

5.

6.

7.

8.

9.

10.

My Top 3 Goals:

1.

2.

3.

It is helpful to use the SMART goal-setting guideline described by Paul J. Meyer in *Attitude is Everything:*

S = Specific	Goals should be clear, concise, detailed, and specific.
M = Measurable	You want to be able to track progress of goals by making them measurable, looking at how much, how many, or how often. Keeping a daily goal log is a great way to track your progress.
A = Action-Oriented	The goal should describe an action-oriented result. What is it that you are going to do to achieve the goal?
R = Realistic & Relevant	Goals should be challenging but realistic, working your way up gradually. They should be achievable so as to not set yourself up for failure.
T = Time-Based	This includes a "by-when" date to help keep you accountable.

Exercise #4: Goal Setting Follow-up Questions

Take some time to reflect on and work through the following questions in your journal:

1. What are the benefits of reaching your goals? What will this get you? Why is this important to you?
2. How will you be affected if you don't reach your goals and never make the change, perpetuating your current habitual patterns? How would that *feel*?
3. How will you be affected if you do reach your goals? How would that *feel*?
4. What are your biggest health risks/dangers? Will achieving your health goals minimize your risk for these health complications?
5. How will you know that you achieved your goals?
6. What are you willing to do to achieve your goals?
7. What help/support do you need to achieve your goals?
8. What can help you be accountable? A journal, a friend, or a support group?
9. How will you celebrate your success on a weekly or monthly basis (that does not include food)?

The Action Plan

The action plan created to support your goals defines how to allocate your time and resources on a day-to-day or week-to-week basis to set yourself up for success. It also allows you to become clear about what responsibility you are willing to take on to make your vision a reality.

Creating an action plan is important because it helps to re-wire your brain to create a new habit, replacing the old habits by keeping your new goals at the forefront of your mind. With a specific action plan that includes details such as when, where, how, with whom, as well as taking note of what you are feeling, you begin to associate these triggers with a new and healthy outcome, prompting you to make the right decisions in alignment with your vision. It can even start to happen spontaneously, outside of your conscious awareness as an automatic response.

For example, as part of your weight-loss goal, you may have the action plan to start each day with a smoothie, at least three mornings per week. This takes a little bit of planning and forward thinking so you're not caught with an empty fridge one morning and more inclined to pick up a coffee and muffin on your way to work. You have to make it easy for yourself so that it becomes an effortless habit. This also means setting a time to go grocery shopping and strategically creating a trigger or cue to remind yourself to make your lunch the night before. You can also use emotions as triggers to prompt you to align with your goals. If you know that a short walk improves your mood and increases the likelihood that you eat healthy, go for a five- to ten-minute walk before you eat lunch. Now you're getting down to the specifics. For example:

- **When + where:** breakfast (7 a.m.) at home.
- **What:** Smoothie. Make a list of three smoothie recipes.
- **How:** Make a list of all the fruits or vegetables that you need and place it on your refrigerator; record it in your agenda or in a smart phone.
- **Another when + where:** Grocery shopping Sunday morning at local farmers market, then grocery store.

Getting specific about your goals is so effective that it also reduces the negative influence that stress, distraction, and fatigue can have on your decision making in the moment you need to make a choice. You're also less likely to fall prey to the negative effects of self-criticism, which sets you up for failure, derailing you from your goals. This process also helps you overcome the common obstacle of simply getting started, allowing you to take the first steps on the path toward your vision.

To give you an idea of what the entire vision, purpose, and goal process looks like on paper, here is an example of the progression from a health vision statement to an underlying purpose statement, followed by goals, with a specific action plan created to achieve those goals:

Health Vision: I see myself at my ideal weight (a realistic *x* number of pounds) and managing my stress more effectively.

Underlying Purpose: Enjoy life, feel better in my body, and enjoy time with loved ones.

Goal #1: Lose 2 pounds per month for a total of 10 pounds by December 1.

Action Plan (behavioral commitments):

- Exercise 3 days/week: Mon/Wed/Fri @ 7 a.m. at the gym. 45 min cardio/25 min core strength class
- At least 2 meals per day consisting of raw fruits and vegetables: Grocery shop twice per week (Sunday & Wednesday), prepare lunch, meal plan for the week

Goal #2: Meditate daily by December 1.

Action Plan (behavioral commitments):

- Sit for 10 minutes at least 3 days per week by October 1.
- Meditate before gym, when I first wake up at 6 a.m.
- Set out meditation cushion the night before.

Planning for Failure

What is going to prevent you from reaching your goals? This may sound like an odd question, but *planning for failure* can actually be as crucial as imagining success. Failing to prepare and plan for obstacles you will inevitably encounter compromises your chances of success.[108] So the next time you go to the movies and you're triggered to walk up and buy popcorn, you have a set plan already in place for what you're going to do instead, like reach into your bag and grab your pre-planned healthy snack. It's important to imagine what will likely be the cause of failure (popcorn at the movies, didn't have time to grocery shop, too tired to work out after work), what obstacles you will face, and what temptations you are likely to give into. Take a moment to close your eyes, and imagine what the scenario will look like, in as much detail as possible.

By going through this process you can initiate what researchers call implementation intentions,[109] which is an if/then plan of action. If x happens (the most likely obstacle I will encounter, such as seeing people eating donuts), then I will do y (go outside for a five-minute walk) to achieve z (my highest goal of optimal health). This strategy helps you to translate your goals into action and gives you some foresight into how you will respond in situations where you're not likely to follow through on your goals.

In one study involving 256 women aged thirty to fifty years old,[110] researchers compared two different interventions to help women increase their physical activity levels. The group of women who were asked to keep track of how they were *not* going to reach their goals, and revise it every day based on what they actually noticed, ended up getting twice as much physical exercise than the group of women who did not practice this technique.

Exercise #5: Planning for Failure

I encourage you to take the time to think about and write down your answers to these questions. This exercise will help you see where you're likely to hit road bumps and plan out what you're going to do about it. Go through this exercise for each of your top three goals.

1. What is your goal?
2. What action will it take to reach this goal?
3. What are the obstacles to reaching this goal? (You can name as many obstacles as necessary. Next to each obstacle outline when and where this obstacle is likely to occur.)
4. What specific action will you take to follow through on your goals when you are facing this specific obstacle?

The Power of Visualization

Do you want to supercharge your efforts with a simple, quick, and, best of all, free technique that you can implement immediately to improve your chances of success? Try visualization. When you visualize yourself making the choice that aligns with your goals, you are activating the same neural networks as if you were actually doing it. Visualization lays the foundation for change so that when the time comes, it's that much easier to make the decision you will be proud of, instead of one you will regret.

The brain doesn't know the difference between current reality and the future memory (also known as "encoding perspective memory") you are creating. So whether you are recalling something you've actually done or imagining something you're going to do, the same part of the brain is activated. In this way, as you visualize yourself engaging in the desired behavioral change, even before it's actually happened, you're strengthening your new habit before you've even done it! The more you imagine yourself doing something, the more likely it is that your brain will automatically do what you've imagined.

There are many benefits to practicing visualization. This practice can help reduce stress and anxiety, improve your focus and attention, boost your mood and self-confidence, and allow you to align with what you want to create in your life. Every single cell in your body "hears" your thoughts: as the famous saying goes: "*as you think, so shall you be.*" As you start to visualize in great detail the state of health you want to manifest, your body will respond.

Visualization requires that you imagine, in as much detail as possible and using all of your senses, what it will be like to experience your desired outcome. One way you can do this is to reread your vision statement and tune into what it *feels* like to be living this vision. Also incorporate into the visualization some part of your routine—for example, waking up and making a healthy smoothie for breakfast. What does your environment look like? What does it feel like to be in your body, to pick up the blender and touch the fruit, to cut it up as you put it into the blender? What does the food smell like? What do you hear? What does it taste like? And how does it feel to be making the healthier choice? Bring the sensory experience alive in your mind's eye. By painting a picture that you can "feel," you're laying the foundation for a healthier lifestyle.

Do you want even better results? Take it one step further and combine visualization with planning for failure: visualize yourself in the situations where you're most likely *not* to follow through on your goals, and then visualize yourself overcoming the obstacle and choosing the best possible course of action.

Pause & Reflect: Assessing Your Readiness for Change

Take a moment to turn your attention inward and assess your readiness for lasting change:

1. Am I motivated to adopt long-term lifestyle changes as opposed to quick-fix solutions?
2. Am I ready to commit to goals to reach my ideal vision of a healthy life?
3. Am I ready to slow down and make time to integrate these new changes in my life?
4. Am I ready to learn more about the benefits of whole foods and commit to my education in this area?
5. Am I ready to become more physically active at least three to four times per week?
6. Am I ready to handle difficult or stressful situations directly, instead of turning to food as a coping mechanism?
7. If I'm in a situation where I don't have access to healthy food choices, am I willing to do my best, stay positive, and not let that one situation spiral me out of control?
8. Am I ready to ask for help when I need support?
9. Am I ready to stop turning to food for support?
10. Am I ready to support myself in other more healthful and loving ways?
11. Am I ready to let go of addictive, hyper-palatable foods and most restaurant food (or seek out healthier restaurant alternatives)?
12. Am I ready to potentially go through possible withdrawal and experience detoxification symptoms?
13. Am I willing to be patient with the weight-loss process and not expect rapid weight loss?
14. Am I ready to look at the underlying reasons, especially emotional and spiritual, that drive me to overeat?
15. Am I ready to let go of food as a means of distraction in my life?
16. Am I ready to become more mindful and conscious of my food choices?
17. Am I willing to look at my food-related patterns without judgment or self-criticism?

Six R's to Unhook Yourself from Your Habitual Food Patterns

One of the biggest obstacles for most people who struggle with food is the difficulty to overcome the impulse to eat in the moment. This is a learned behavioral response that is an ingrained and unconscious habit. Use the six R's as a powerful process for overcoming food addiction, compulsive overeating, and cravings for hyper-palatable foods—foods that have no place in your new, healthy lifestyle.

1. **Recognize.** Become aware of your cues and triggers. Start to recognize where you are and what you see, smell, or think right before you feel the overwhelming urge to eat. What time of day is it? Who are you with? What were you feeling right before you were triggered? If you can't identify your trigger, simply notice what is coming up for you and what you are feeling in the present moment.

2. **Reframe.** This requires a drastic shift in perception. Look at the processed hyper-palatable food for what it really is: refined sugar layered on top of fat, on top of more refined sugar, on top of more fat, topped with a lot of salt. Look at it as addiction, struggle, or a heart attack on a plate—look at it as disgusting. Whatever works for you. Once you know the truth about something, perceptions change. Ask yourself: do I want to put this in my body?

3. **Remember.** Remember what it feels like to be hooked on this food, and feel the struggle that goes along with it. Remember your rock-bottom moment. Remember the pain inherent in eating this way. Do you want to perpetuate that cycle? How do you feel right after you eat this? How long does that feeling last for and affect you? Hours? Days? Weeks?

4. **Reconnect.** Take a moment and reconnect in your heart with the millions of other people who also struggle in this way, a self-compassionate act that connects you to our shared humanity. You can remember to connect to others by setting an aspiration like: "May we all be free of suffering." By remembering your connection to others, you immediately foster compassion, a powerful tool to unhook yourself from the urges of the present moment.

5. **Refocus.** When you notice yourself getting caught up in your struggle with food, don't forget to step back and paint your "bigger picture" perspective by focusing on the bigger vision of your ideal healthy future. Ask yourself if eating what you are about to eat is in alignment with your health-related vision and the goals you've set. (And remember that sometimes you may

consciously choose to eat something that's not in alignment with your goals; in this case, since you are choosing it, don't feel bad about it! Be mindful of the experience of eating and be open to what it may teach you about future food choices.)

6. **Rotate.** This is where you actively *choose* the reality with which you want to align. Turn around and focus your attention on something else. Play music, lie outside on the grass and get some sun, read a good book, light some candles and take a nice relaxing bath. Choose any healthy activity that will help you to feel good in this moment.

Self-Compassion: Especially During Relapse

When it comes to making health-related changes, you can expect challenges, you can expect difficult times—heck, you can probably even count on lapses and relapses. If you berate yourself for doing something that wasn't in alignment with your goals, you will certainly and ultimately have a harder time in reaching them. Learn to navigate these challenging moments with self-compassion and confidence. If you've done something that wasn't in alignment with your values and goals, you can tap into self-kindness, a key component of self-compassion, to help steer yourself back onto the path you'd rather be on. It's not merely saying that whatever just happened is *okay* or *fine* (see self-criticism versus self-indulgence, chapter 5); it's acknowledging that what you just did doesn't serve your highest purpose, intentions, or values, and hasn't met your deepest needs, and now it's time to put one foot in front of the other in the direction that lines up with your heartfelt desires.

When we practice self-compassion, we learn to drop unnecessary layers of suffering. When feeling depressed, for example, we can practice self-compassion. At the first signs of depression, instead of fueling further depression with self-criticism and harsh judgments, we can learn to stay with the underlying quality or energy of what we're feeling and accept it and even welcome it in with love, compassion, and non-judgment.

Making Friends with Yourself

One of the keys to achieving your health goals is to fully acknowledge and accept where you are right now and start from there. This often requires a healthy dose of self-compassion. When you think about it, despite how much you may resist it—what other choice do you have but to start where you already are? But how often do you wish that you could start someplace else—anywhere but right here? Wouldn't you rather start ten pounds lighter or at least in a better mood, or maybe wait until Monday morning? If you simply acknowledge and accept where you currently are, in a non-judgmental way, then you can consciously choose whether you want to stay there or move in the direction of a happier, healthier lifestyle—one step at a time.

Pause & Reflect: Making Friends with Yourself

Take a moment to reflect on the following questions:

1. Have you been trying, struggling, and pushing to "get over there" (ten pounds thinner, more energetic, etc.) because you don't love yourself exactly as you are?
2. Are you ready to love and accept yourself now, just as you are?
3. Do you feel worthy of living a healthy, happy life?

Accepting where you're starting from requires a willingness to make friends with yourself, exactly as you are.* If you have the willingness and courage to see that you have gained weight this year, to accept it without judgment and self-criticism, and then move forward from a place of loving-kindness, you greatly improve your chances of stepping off the roller coaster all together and establishing fundamental changes to your health. However, if your desire for change is rooted in self-rejection of who you are in this present moment, actually maintaining positive, lasting change will prove to be more difficult. If you reject yourself because you think you weigh too much, then you're likely to still have underlying self-resentment after you lose the weight. You have not actually made friends with who you are, no matter what you look like. Practicing self-acceptance is a fundamental part of self-compassion and is a good place to start.

Fostering self-acceptance is rooted in the belief that you are worthy of living a healthier, happier life. You deserve to step onto this path where you are free of your struggle with food and your weight and where you feel amazing in your body. When you choose to feel good now, or at least be open and curious about whatever you may be feeling, you choose to drop the struggle; as a secondary result of living from this heart space of genuinely feeling good, you're also more likely to drop the

---

* This concept of "making friends with yourself" was first introduced to me many years ago by one of my most cherished teachers, Pema Chödrön.

weight—naturally. Weight loss becomes a natural byproduct of feeling good, not the centralized focus.

Exercise #6: Developing Self-Compassion: Be There for a Friend

A great way to practice the qualities of self-compassion (the mindful observer, kindness, and common humanity) is to imagine a friend coming to you with the difficult situation you currently find yourself to be in. What would you say to your friend? What kind of tone would you use to comfort them? Perhaps you would console them with words of encouragement and remind them that everyone goes through hard times; it's part of being human. Notice how this support for your friend is rooted in gentleness, patience, and kindness. Notice how you empathize with their suffering with a sense of open attentiveness. Pay attention to how you maintain your own level of emotional poise and stability without getting swept away or lost in emotional reactions. There's no judgment, and you're not trying to change the situation for you or them; you're just supporting them through this process. Take a moment to pause. Now shift your focus back to you and your situation and apply that same level of compassionate support to yourself.

It's the Path, Not the Destination

I use the term "health goals" quite frequently in this chapter, but it is important to remember that this is a journey and to take joy in the fact that you are now on the path, aspiring for better health. Relax and loosen your grip on the concept of *rigidly* defined goals. Yes, it is important to have goals, but you can also become obsessed with reaching them and thinking that if you don't, you are doomed to failure. When you become fixated on some imaginary time in the future, you miss out on the precious "now" of your life. That is not the intention here. The word "goal" is already so imbued with relentless striving; perhaps, instead, we should say health *aspiration*. In this way, we aspire to be healthier, but with a softer, more accepting stance. Find the balance between "too rigid" and "too loose" that is most suitable for you.

Embarking on a healthier lifestyle is not like taking a one-way express ticket to your final destination. Everything is always in motion, constantly changing, and learning to embrace these fluctuations will surely aid you on this journey.

In relation to weight loss, it's not a straight line where you keep losing until you reach your desired weight. Perhaps one of your health aspirations is to learn to be okay with that. When you have a hard time accepting the fluctuations, it's easier to give up at the first sight of failure. I'm sure you've experienced this; I know I have.

> "This too is a pervasive tragedy . . . that we might miss the actuality of the life that is ours to live because we are so distracted, preoccupied, and driven by attempting to attain some mind-constructed ideal in some other time that is often also, sadly, shaped by unexamined desires, aversions, and illusions."
>
> —Jon Kabat-Zinn, from the foreword of
> Jan Chozen Bays' *Mindful Eating*

When you are too harsh with yourself and have high expectations, usually ones that are unattainable or unsustainable, you set yourself up for failure. This is at the root of the well-known starting/stopping, striving/flopping, on/off mentality. You find yourself on an emotional roller coaster of "I can do it/I can't do it, I'm losing/I'm gaining, I'm good/I'm bad, I'm on the wagon/I'm off the wagon." Do you see what I mean? When I go out for a run, I no longer set rigidly defined expectations of myself. I know the direction I want to go in, I encourage myself to do the best I can, and I also honor my body's needs and know that living in this body is a different and new experience each and every day. When I used to tell myself "I need to run the whole way in less than this amount of time" I would often get overwhelmed or stop running when I realized I couldn't reach my goal. That level of "rigidity" was not helpful to me, so I learned to adopt a softer stance to maintain my motivation to put on my running shoes again the next day. I found a balance point that works for me, and I encourage you to explore what that looks like for you. I also remind myself to have fun and bring a playful attitude to the goals I set and remember that staying positive and happy is of prime importance to me.

Now that I am able to take a more gentle approach with myself, I'm not always either "on" or "off" the wagon. When I'm feeling down on myself, I take a more compassionate approach, which allows me to just keep on going. This is not to be confused with not caring; in fact, it's about caring very deeply. We learn to genuinely want what's right for us—without the dead weight of self-criticism and rigid thinking holding us down.

When we learn to be gentler with ourselves, we see our weekly fluctuations no longer as high mountains and low valleys. Instead they become more like the scenic rolling hills of life. This is freedom.

Off the Hook

You have the power to create new habits; ones that serve you and the highest vision you hold for yourself. Stress and self-criticism are like strapping a dead weight to your motivation and forces your brain to revert to those old habitual cycles you're trying not to perpetuate. How you behave is shaped and driven by how you think and which part of the mind—conscious or unconscious—is being activated. As we will see in the next part of this book, the reason many people overeat is strongly linked to their mental state of mind. How you choose to engage with "mindfulness" will play a key role in strengthening the conscious part of your mind, reinforcing new behavioral patterns, and slowly but surely helping you end your struggle with food.

PART FOUR

The Mental Hook

"To end our struggle, we must learn to not let regret, worry, or fear dominate our life in the present moment. Each minute we spend worrying about the future and regretting the past is a minute we miss in our appointment with life—a missed opportunity to engage life and to see that each moment gives us a chance to change for the better, to experience peace and joy."

—**Thich Nhat Hanh,** *Savor: Mindful Eating, Mindful Life*

Chapter 7

How Our
Mental State Hooks Us

I remember this scenario from my past all too well: I'd be eating a bag of chips in front of the television, and before I knew it, I would look down and the bag was empty. Had I really eaten that whole bag? I would look suspiciously at my sister, but she was sitting too far away to reach. If you're not present while eating, does it count as eating? Unfortunately, the calories definitely count, just as they count when you're eating the chocolate cake standing in front of the fridge with the door open, while no one was looking. Not only the calories count, but also the lack of nourishment you feel from not paying attention—as it turns out, it counts quite a lot.

We live in a highly distracted, three-second attention span culture, where we're constantly on autopilot, going through the repetitive motions of the day . . . brush teeth, drive to work, grab a coffee, watch TV . . . without being aware of what's actually happening in the present moment. This behavior is driven by our automatic mind, as introduced in chapter 5, and can also be referred to as *mindlessness*. As we discussed, the automatic mind is the part of the brain that governs habitual patterns, especially surrounding survival-based mechanisms like eating. Simply put, we overeat because we're not paying attention! While on autopilot, we do the same thing we've done a thousand times, we're not paying attention to what we're doing and instead, we're lost in a completely unrelated train of thought. When we're not fully present in the moment but instead are distracted in la-la land, we are experiencing mindlessness. Combine mindlessness with eating, and what do we get? Overeating. As a result we miss the opportunity to connect to the special gift inherent in food that *mindfulness* can offer us.

"When we are able to fully appreciate the basic activities of eating and drinking, we discover an ancient secret, the secret of how to become content and at ease."

Jan Chozen Bays, *Mindful Eating*

Mindlessness

Although the word "mindlessness" might make you think of a mind that's *not* thinking, it's actually the complete opposite. In fact, mindlessness usually means that we're swept away by the tides of our thoughts. We're lost in thought rather than *experiencing* what we're doing in the "now" through awareness of our senses and surroundings. Yes, we do have moments when we "zone out" and little mental activity takes place, yet this is the exception rather than the rule in our busy lives. We are mindless when we are:

- Rushing from place to place
- Absentminded
- Habitually reacting rather than responding to situations
- Worrying about the future
- Focusing on the past
- Judging our experiences with guilt, blame, or fear
- Wanting or craving for more
- Obsessing over material possessions
- Avoiding unpleasant sensations and feelings
- Resisting what we are feeling in the moment
- Out of touch with our body and not listening to what it is telling us

Now, reread the list and notice that an extremely busy mind and incessant thinking usually accompany all of these mindless activities.

When I share this list at workshops and ask how many people have experienced any one of these in the last twenty-four hours, the group always laughs—it's funny because it's sad, but true. Most people experience some or all of these as a regular part of their day, on an hourly basis. If you identify with any one of these on the list, join the club. Most people live in a near constant state of mindlessness and ongoing, endless thinking about almost everything else other than what they are actually doing.

Mindlessness Applied to Eating

Because we eat every day, we tend to create habitual patterns around eating, which usually develops into mindless eating. As a result, we lose the special experience that food can offer us. As a culture we are constantly on the go, and many people feel they don't have time to sit down to eat. People eat in a rush—while walking, standing, driving, watching TV, talking on the phone, or sitting at the computer— and forget to pay attention, let alone enjoy the food being eaten. When you eat with distractions and don't pay attention to what you're eating, you're more likely to be left feeling unsatisfied, creating a cycle of overeating.

Pause & Reflect: What Is Your Experience with Mindless Eating?

Take a moment to think about how often you have experienced the "bottom of the bag" syndrome. What were you doing while you were eating? How do you normally eat? Standing up at the counter? Sitting at your desk at work in front of the computer? How about in front of the TV? Do you ever eat so fast you wonder where it went or what it even tasted like?

Mindlessness impacts how we experience eating and how we experience food, and by extension how we experience life. When was the last time you sat down and fully enjoyed a nourishing meal without any distractions?

Effects of Mindless Eating—Starving the Spirit

When we eat mindlessly, we can't truly appreciate or enjoy our food. We don't allow ourselves to savor the pleasure of eating and to really taste what we are eating, and many times we are left still feeling hungry. The hunger is not necessarily physical hunger, especially not after unconsciously overeating, but a sort of "wanting" is left within us. We feel dissatisfied, unfulfilled, and disconnected from the experience of eating, and even though we may no longer be hungry, we still *want* more. Have you ever experienced that? Have you ever wondered why that is? It's because food does not only nourish us physically. When we eat mindfully and with gratitude, we nourish ourselves not only physically, but emotionally, mentally, and spiritually as well.

> **"If we want to feel satisfied as we eat, the mind has to be aware of what is occurring in the mouth. In other words, if you want to have a party in your mouth, the mind has to be invited."**
>
> —Jan Chozen Bays, *Mindful Eating*

Impact of Mindless Eating

There are very real and physical consequences to engaging with our food mindlessly:

- **Loss of ability to detect physical hunger and satiety.** Dieting, overeating, and suppressing hunger strongly inhibit awareness of the natural body rhythms and internal body awareness of knowing when the body is hungry and when it is full.
- **Weight gain.** Lack of attention and autopilot behavior can trigger excess food consumption.
- **Nutritional deficiencies**. When not tuning into what your *body* needs and wants, you may instead be feeding it foods that it does not recognize, such as processed, refined foods. This can lead to excess calorie intake, yet still starve your body of required essential nutrients.
- **Digestive distress**. When you eat in a rush or in a state of stress, less blood tends to flow to your stomach to aid digestion. This can cause digestive distress and uncomfortable symptoms like gas and bloating.

The ultimate effect of mindless eating is a feeling of discontent. This may trigger you to spiral down a path of dissatisfaction with yourself and with food and lead to the familiar self-centered struggle with food and weight. When caught in this space of struggling, food becomes a distraction, making it more difficult to focus on what your life is truly about: living your joy and purpose. Because food becomes a source of your struggling, you allow it to hold you down rather than lift you up and propel you forward, and you lose the connection to the miracle food truly is: divine energy for your life's journey.

What Is Mindfulness?

Mindfulness is an ancient solution to healthy living and is proving to be the much-needed antidote to the chaotic state of our food environment discussed in chapter 1 and the mindless eating that accompanies it. Mindfulness is the practice of being fully present—here, now. Mindfulness is the doorway through which you can end your struggle with your weight. If you choose, once you walk through this doorway of mindfulness and commit to embarking on this path, you will see everything in a new light; your life will no longer be what it was. When you choose to focus on living a mindful life, you are choosing to come home to yourself and wake up to this miracle called life.

Mindfulness is a very simple tool that can produce profound results. The more mindful we become, the more enriched and full our lives will be. Mindfulness disengages our habitual reactive behaviors and allows for inner wisdom to emerge. It strengthens our prefrontal cortex (PFC), the part of the brain related to insight and higher-order decision-making. Mindfulness also strengthens your willpower and allows you to focus on your goals, and the bigger picture of what you want your life to become. This is a powerful part of the brain to tap into and can serve you well on your journey to health and total freedom from the struggle with food.

Mindfulness Means Experiencing What Is

Chronic distraction is part of our culture. This includes distracting ourselves from emotions. We don't want to feel what we're feeling because it might not feel good, so we pick up the remote, we open the fridge door, we go online or go shopping, or we reach for the cigarette, the joint, the pill or the alcohol. Not wanting to feel what we are feeling is the root of most addictions. We all have some level of addiction to something, even if it's very subtle. Traditional wisdom holds that mindfulness is actually our natural state of being; we've just been practicing and strengthening our methods of distraction for so long we've drifted further and further away from this truth. Although we may reach for things to distract ourselves and satisfy our addictions unconsciously, we all have the capability to become more mindful of our actions, and we all can learn to strengthen our "mindfulness muscles" with a commitment to practice.

Although it may sound counterintuitive, mindfulness occurs when we learn to quiet our incessant, distracted thoughts (aka monkey mind) and instead have a direct experience with what we are doing in the present moment. Mindfulness is awareness, not necessarily thinking, which are two different things. Mindfulness is about being present to each moment, as each moment is a totally new experience—one that never happened before and will never happen again. It's about being aware of what you're experiencing through your senses, your breath, and your surroundings—both your inner and outer environment. Feeling the sun on your face without needing to think, "I love the sun on my face, the sun feels so good, I should get out and do this more often, I wonder if I'm burning . . . " Mindfulness allows you to simply *be*, to experience the present moment without the need to label or define that experience.

Mindfulness can also involve noticing what you're feeling and staying with that feeling, no matter how bad it feels—not distracting yourself away from it (usually through unhealthy habitual patterns of distraction). Mindfulness also means that you become aware of the thoughts you're thinking, the thoughts that keep coming and going like a never-ending movie, without necessarily believing them or attaching to them, but simply noticing, like witnessing a series of clouds passing by.

Jon Kabat-Zinn, a world-renowned mindfulness and meditation teacher, defines mindfulness as "paying attention, on purpose, in a particular way."

This is a very simple statement with much depth to it, so let's look at it more closely. What are we paying attention *to*? Mindfulness allows us to pay attention to how we live our lives on a moment-by-moment basis. If we spend most of our time thinking about the future or dwelling on the past, we're going to miss out on our entire lives—all the little intricacies and tiny miracles that make up the sum of our experience. The message is about focusing your awareness on whatever you choose to focus on—whatever is currently happening in the present moment.

"On purpose" refers to the intention that we set—setting the *intention to pay attention*—and how engaged we are in the process. The last part, "in a particular way," is *how* we choose to pay attention, the attitude we show up with. Think of it as the mood or tone surrounding our mindfulness practice. The attitudes of mindfulness practice include:

- Acceptance and non-judgment
- Openness and a willingness to stay with whatever thoughts or feelings arise
- Deep trust in the process as our experience unfolds on a moment-to-moment basis

- Fearlessness in the face of whatever arises
- Kindness, compassion, and gentleness for ourselves and others
- Non-striving, just being where you are with the knowing that you have already arrived
- Patience and calmness
- Letting go of attachment to the outcome
- A sense of lightheartedness and humor

These are the qualities worth fostering. They help us feel good about ourselves and the world we live in, and soften our hearts towards ourselves and those around us.

When we understand that we all have the capacity to be mindful, we can take this awareness and apply it to mindful eating. Although it may be a slow practice, there are many benefits from learning to eat mindfully. Paying attention to the present moment, on a moment-by-moment basis, is the antidote to an unhealthy and addictive relationship with food; it's not only what you eat but how and why you eat.

Mindfulness Applied to Eating

We can now take everything we've learned about mindfulness and apply it to eating. When you learn to become mindful of what, when, where, how much, and with whom you eat, it activates your conscious mind and helps create lasting, positive change to your relationship with food: you gain greater awareness, you develop loving acceptance, and you take mindful action in the direction of your new and healthier future.

"Awareness and compulsion cannot coexist, since the latter depends on the obliteration of the former."

—**Geneen Roth,** *Women Food and God*

Take Heart: Mindfulness Is Worth the Commitment

It isn't always easy to become aware. Maybe you're thinking, "Who possibly has the time to be mindful of every single bite? I need to constantly multitask just to keep up with my life!" It takes a certain level of practice and dedication to foster the wonderful gift of mindfulness. It also forces you to "wake up," and if you've been unaware for a long time, it may not be easy to actually look at yourself and the habits you've developed over the years.

Mindful eating can shake you out of habitual patterns that may be very comforting to you, ones that you've grown to rely on for support, but at what cost to your life and your health? The path of mindfulness encourages you to look at what you're actually doing, why you are eating when you're not hungry, and to face your distractions. These are not easy issues to deal with, but on the other side of the struggle, if you are brave enough to work through it instead of burying it with food, what you will find is space, and in that space you will find freedom of choice. In chapter 10, we will look at a basic mediation practice and how you can use simple techniques to work with your emotions and feel what you're feeling, instead of using food as a way to cope or distract.

> "If we are always on the way to someplace else, to some better now, when we will be thinner, or happier, or more accomplished, or whatever it is, then we can never be in wise relationship with this moment and love ourselves as we actually are."
>
> —Jon Kabat-Zinn

Top Ten Benefits of Mindful Eating

When we bring mindful awareness to the eating process, the experience of eating looks and feels very different from what you may be accustomed to. There are many benefits of committing to the mindful path, but the real work we need to do in order to grow as a human being is not always easy. With focused effort, you too can reap the many benefits of learning to eat more mindfully.

These are just a few of the ways that mindful eating can improve your relationship with food, to your body, to the earth, and to life itself:

1. **Discover the power of choice.** How many times have you felt that overeating was beyond your control, as if you had no choice? Mindfulness allows you to instantly create a space between the desire to eat and the act of eating. Mindful eating interrupts the impulse, the automatic pilot you've become habituated to, and creates a moment of space where you can be present enough to make a conscious choice.

2. **Eat based on internal cues.** By continuously checking in with your inner and outer reality, mindful eating can allow you to be guided by your internal body awareness. By using the mindful eating tools presented in chapter 8, you will become more attuned to your internal cues of hunger and satiety

by pausing and tuning in, and you will be able to ask yourself, "Am I still hungry?"

3. **Develop trust in yourself.** Do you ever feel like you just can't trust yourself around food? Perhaps you've flexed your "give-in" muscle one too many times and have created a habit of eating impulsively. Practicing mindful eating tunes you into your own inherent wisdom, and teaches you to trust yourself to make the right decisions about your body's needs. This leads to improved self-awareness and increases your resiliency toward the challenges of life.

4. **Sustain a healthy weight.** Weight management becomes easier as you learn to put down the fork before you feel stuffed. Through this process, you allow your mind to step out of the way and use your internal cues to guide you to optimal weight levels. When you feel present with what you're eating, you also feel more nourished and satisfied. This is a key element to sustaining a positive relationship with food and subsequent weight management.

5. **Create brighter moods and more energy.** Overeating can often leave us feeling sluggish. This is because digestion requires a lot of physical energy. When you slow down and listen to your internal cues, you can stop eating before you get too full, and you will not waste so much of your precious energy on digestion, freeing up your energy to focus on other things in your life.

6. **Improve mental capacities**. Through the process of neuroplasticity, mindfulness helps restructure your brain in new ways and has been linked to increased mental clarity, improved working memory, and focus.

7. **Address food issues at their source**. This is the crux of what mindful eating is all about for most people. You learn to address the root or underlying cause of what you are actually feeling instead of stuffing your feelings down with food.

8. **Offers you an abundance mentality**. If you're like most people, you may have a difficult time leaving food on your plate, or you may suffer from a "food-lack mentality," dutifully eating (with guilt) to avoid wasting food. This particular group of people tends to belong to the "Clean Your Plate Club." Mindful eating encourages you to address these issues at their source, reminds you that we live in food abundance, and that we can share that abundance with others, opening up a space of generosity within ourselves, countering any food "hoarding" mentality that we may have.

9. **Learn to truly enjoy food.** When you focus on the miracle that each bite holds for you—instead of the TV show you're watching—you can gain a deep sense of pleasure from eating, creating an enjoyable, relaxed experience around food.

10. **Deepen your connection to the sacred.** Mindful eating is about becoming aware of the connectedness that everything shares. You can change your entire relationship with food when you connect to its source. Your perception shifts to one of deep gratitude because food—real food—is such a miracle!

"Mindful eating also has the unexpected benefits of helping us tap into our body's natural wisdom and our heart's natural capacity for openness and gratitude."

—**Jan Chozen Bays,** *Mindful Eating*

Getting Unhooked

Although you may have been conditioning yourself to eat mindlessly for many years, you can learn to eat more mindfully, one bite at a time. When you take the time to slow things down around the eating process and tune in, you're able to appreciate the abundance that nature offers you. Eating mindfully allows you to feel satisfied, to feel nurtured by and connected to the earth. It allows you to realize the gifts that are right in front of you and foster gratitude and appreciation for these gifts, allowing you to honor the food you eat and thus honor yourself. It's these core essential benefits that result in weight loss, increased energy, clear skin, stable moods, and other physical, emotional, mental and spiritual improvements—natural byproducts of living and eating mindfully.

Chapter 8

Unhooked: Learning to Eat Mindfully

Mindful eating is simple and subtle, yet profound and powerful. It's not exactly something that you can quantify, measure, or dissect with your intellect. I invite you to let your analytical mind step aside and allow your *experience* to guide you. The guidelines presented in this chapter are merely a roadmap to what will eventually be your own direct experience to uncovering the miracle of food through mindfulness. In order to gain the many benefits of mindful eating, you need to take the time to practice. I will point you in the right direction and shed light on the extraordinary power of incorporating mindful eating into your life, but at the end of the day, only practice will bring you closer to experiencing the exquisite gift of the present moment.

"You are learning a new language now. In this process, your body is your best friend and most important teacher. You must learn to honour it once more, to not denigrate or distrust it as you have been taught in school. It knows and will teach you. If you let it. If you respect it."

—Stephen Harrod Buhner

If you're looking for a mindless quick-fix solution to weight loss, then you're in the wrong place—or at least the wrong book. The practice of mindfulness, especially applied to eating, is a lifelong daily practice, one that's worth every single moment of time you're willing to dedicate to it. I'm reminded of what my guitar teacher used to say to encourage me to keep practicing: "Slow and steady wins the race." This has truth to it. We all repeatedly come to that moment that feels like a fork in the road (pun intended) where we have a choice: to wake up to our highest selves through mindful awareness, or to repeat the automatic habitual patterns that we know cause us suffering. You can walk this mindful path, awakening to your inner wisdom, one slow and steady step at a time, eventually opening like a beautiful flower, or you can keep going round and round with your old habitual patterns of eating and living unconsciously, contributing to your unhappiness. The path you choose is up to you, but the mindful path requires that you continuously keep choosing it, each and every day. Even though it feels like you're only inching along, over time you will look back and see how far you've actually come.

Slow Down

The first thing people usually think about when I say mindful eating is "slooooooow motion." Although mindfulness does not necessarily mean slow, slowing down is a helpful practice, as you have more time to notice and observe what you're doing. You can almost hear your mom's voice in your head nagging you to "chew your food." Mom's got a point on this one. It's essential that we learn to slow down the eating process. This not only allows us to actually taste, savor, and enjoy our food, but it also gives us time to register how full we are. A lot of overeating happens simply because we eat too much too fast, without giving our brain enough time to recognize that we're full and to send the appropriate messages back to the body to stop eating.

Eating slowly is a simple and highly effective method to prevent overeating. The research speaks for itself. New studies by the University of Rhode Island[111] have found that heavier people eat faster than slimmer people. Other research conducted at Osaka University in Japan studied the eating habits of three thousand people. They found that men who ate quickly were 84 percent more likely to be overweight, and women were twice as likely to be overweight as the slower eaters.

If you're trying to reach your weight-loss goals, eating slowly allows enough time for the appetite-related hormones to kick in and let your brain know you've had enough. When you're eating with others, try to eat as slow or slower than the slowest eater at the table. You can also practice slowing down by setting your fork down between bites, taking more time to chew your food, eating with your non-dominant hand, or eating with chopsticks.

"I don't think it takes more time to be mindful than it takes to be mindless."

—Myla Kabat-Zinn

The REAL Food Approach to Mindful Eating

In the mindful eating workshops that I host in Hawaii, I lead people through a mindfulness exercise. I ask participants to pick an orange right from the tree, where they have a chance to connect to their food source, and I guide them through a mindful eating process defined later in this chapter. It sounds incredibly simple, yet after going through this practice many people make comments such as "I can't believe I'd never really tasted an orange before!" or "Wow, eating *is* deeply spiritual," or "I realize how often I eat when I'm not hungry." It's amazing to see how this process helps us to address and uncover our underlying relationship with food and why we eat the way we do.

Exercise #1: Last Bite of Your Life

Imagine that a doctor told you that you were about to lose the functioning of your taste buds and that you had one meal left to fully taste and experience. How would you interact with that meal? Would you scarf it down, or be fully present to experience every single sensation, reaping the full pleasure and enjoyment that this food had to offer? Would you take the time to feast on it through your eyes? Would you use your sense of smell first? Do you think you would savor it more, exploring the textures and tasting it more fully?

We usually don't appreciate what we have until we don't have it anymore. How do you think this exercise will change the way you taste your next bite of food?

I developed the REAL Food Approach to Mindful Eating as an easy way for people to remember to eat more mindfully. Most people habitually fall back into automatic pilot and the primary reason people don't practice is simply because they forget! This is an invitation to reconnect to the pleasure of eating from a non-compulsive and balanced perspective. We don't have to struggle with food. Eating real food can be a great pleasure and gift, but only if we're present to experience and appreciate it. Besides REAL referring to eating *real* food—one of my most important guidelines to healthy nutrition—it also stands for:

- Relax
- Evaluate
- Awareness
- Loving-kindness

I can't promise you that this practice will always be pleasant or easy. Sometimes it might be quite challenging and uncomfortable, as you uncover underlying emotions or habitual patterns that you may have been covering over with food. If you stay committed to incorporating this mindful approach into the everyday reality of your life, you will notice a huge difference in the way you relate to food, to your body, and to the earth—and recognize them as the miracles they are.

Practice Makes Perfect

I encourage you to start practicing these mindful eating techniques in "easier" environments—situations without a lot of triggers and distractions—so you can have the space to practice tuning in, and then apply them to the more challenging situations (hello social events). Start by practicing this at home in a quiet environment, either alone or with one other person. You may want to let your eating companion know that you're practicing mindful eating and invite them to join you; they may benefit from this process as well.

If you're feeling courageous and want to try this at a family event or holiday, by all means jump on in. But don't get discouraged if old patterns emerge; just stick with the practice and remind yourself to keep coming back to the present moment. No matter the circumstance, it's always beneficial to become more aware of your eating patterns so you can help change them.

Creating Space, Creating Choice

Think of the REAL Food Approach as a technique that acts as a safety speed bump to eating. Think about the last time you were triggered to eat and you ate out of impulse. Can you remember what this impulse felt like in your body? If you can take a moment to pause and explore this impulse or urge to eat, then you might notice an energy or force underlying this impulse; this is the energy of craving and desire. Watch out, because as I'm sure you already know, it can build up and take over really fast. Mindfulness helps to interrupt that momentum. This is the essence of these mindful eating practices: it allows you to pause for long enough in order for you to gain awareness and insight into the choices you're making —no judgment, just noticing. It allows you to create a brief pause between you and your food, between the *desire* to eat and the *act* of eating, so that you can insert conscious choice into the equation. You always have the freedom to choose, but only when you are in a conscious, mindful state. At first the pause between wanting to eat and actually eating might be ever so slight, a tiny sliver of a new reality, but with practice, this space to choose will widen, and you will find yourself in a more peaceful place, where working with desire becomes more manageable.

R = Relax

We live in a culture where there is an incessant need to constantly be *doing*. In our fast-paced lives, we live under unrealistic time pressures and expectations. Stress is now so commonplace, many people have forgotten how to simply take a moment to rest and relax.

There are many good reasons to pause and relax before you eat. Research has discovered that taking a few moments to practice mindful awareness prior to eating can indeed affect the way you digest and metabolize food and its impact on your health.[112]

Cortisol Impairs Digestion

When you eat in a rush, you may be activating the "fight or flight" response in your body, releasing a stress hormone into your system called cortisol. When cortisol increases, digestion automatically decreases. When you eat in a state of anxiety (stress), there is less blood flow to your stomach to aid the digestive process. This can cause digestive distress and can result in gas, bloating, burping, and stomach pain, leading to poor digestion that results in a lack of nutrient absorption, decreased satiety, and overeating.

Breathing Through Your Nose

According to the yogic traditions, the mouth is for eating and the nose for breathing. Breathing through your nose rather than your mouth has a number of advantages, including filtering, warming, and humidifying the air before it enters the lungs. This activates a different biological response than breathing through your mouth. Breathing through your nose tends to activate your parasympathetic nervous system (PSNS) while breathing through your mouth tends to activate your sympathetic nervous system (SNS). Why does this matter? The parasympathetic and sympathetic nervous systems typically function in opposition to each other. The sympathetic nervous system prepares us for the "fight or flight" response in the face of perceived danger. For our ancestors (or for those of us living and spending time in the wilderness), coming across a big bear would activate the sympathetic nervous system. This induces a stress response, a set of physiological responses in the body that includes cortisol release. In today's world we are constantly being triggered by perceived stress that stimulates our sympathetic nervous systems. The PSNS acts to calm down and reverse SNS stimulation by slowing heart rate and regulating digestion, among other things.

"Breathing in and out through the nose helps us take fuller, deeper breaths, which stimulates the lower lung to distribute greater amounts of oxygen throughout the body. Also, the lower lung is rich with the parasympathetic nerve receptors associated with calming the body and mind, whereas the upper lungs — which are stimulated by chest and mouth breathing — prompt us to hyperventilate and trigger sympathetic nerve receptors, which result in the fight or flight reaction."

—**Gwen Lawrence**

Slowing down, centering yourself, and taking time to relax into the present moment, as well as breathing through your nose, can help initiate the activation of your PSNS. This will allow you to eat in a peaceful state and help improve digestion and assimilation of your food. This is one of the easiest ways to help you tune into mindful eating.

Mealtime Relaxation Tips

Here are a couple of tips to help you slow down and activate your PSNS:

1. Close your eyes and take three deep, even breaths through your nose, releasing any tension from your body. Notice your heart rate slowing down. If you feel any shortness of breath, keep focusing on your breath and

breathing through your nose. Let go of all the activities that led you to this point in your day. Take your time here. Even if you feel like you don't have a lot of time for this meal, give yourself permission to make your health a top priority in this moment.

2. Make a conscious effort to connect to a thought that makes you feel good. Feeling good also helps initiate the relaxation response. Think of something you're grateful for, like the food in front of you or the last kind act you witnessed; think of someone who made you smile, or think of your favorite place in the world. Find that soft spot in your heart that feels good. Welcome the relaxation response into that space. Rest here for a few moments.

E = Evaluate

The second step in the REAL Food Approach to Mindful Eating is to *evaluate* your physical hunger. Although it seems like there are hundreds of different reasons why we eat, we can group all of them into two general categories: because we're hungry or because we're cued or triggered to eat—with a myriad of possibilities falling under the latter category. If you can train yourself to check in and evaluate your hunger level every time you are about to eat—whether it's following an impulse or sitting down to a pleasant meal—you will soon realize how often you are driven to eat despite being hungry. At this point, you can then open a doorway of awareness as to *why* you're eating when you're not hungry and look at what is actually driving your hunger.

> "By definition, eating compulsively is eating without regard to the body's cues; it therefore follows that when you develop the capacity to steer your attention back to your body, are aware of what it says, and are willing to listen to it, compulsion falls away."
>
> —**Geneen Roth**, *Women Food and God*

Use these tools to evaluate what you *really* need when you're not hungry so you can learn how to meet those needs without food. When you're willing to look at what you do habitually, you can finally stop adding the many layers of self-sabotage and coping strategies that aren't helping and are only making things worse.

Part of this process is learning how to decipher between internal and external cues. In the first chapter we talked about external cues in our environment that trigger us to eat when we're not hungry. Luckily, we also have internal cues that let us know when we are hungry, when to start and stop eating. These cues are rooted in our physiological intelligence; mindfulness can teach you how to favor your internal cues based on actual hunger rather than external cues based on craving, impulse, and unconscious triggers. We can also be triggered to eat based on non-hunger related internal cues, like our thoughts and emotions, which we will discuss in Part Five. For the purpose of the following discussion, we are referring to our hunger-related internal cues.

Internal Versus External Cues

Author Brian Wansink found that normal-weight people indicated they were more likely to be influenced by internal cues of meal cessation, while overweight people indicated they were more influenced by external cues.[113] He conducted a very interesting study with two groups of people: from Paris and from Boston. What he found was that the French were influenced by internal cues of meal cessation, while Americans were more influenced by external cues. When asked a series of questions concerning how they knew it was time to stop eating, the French typically answered the question "I usually stop eating when . . ." based on internal cues, such as:

- "I start feeling full."
- "I want to leave room for dessert."
- "If it doesn't taste good, I'll still eat it if I am hungry." (In other words, they are eating based on actual hunger and less based on taste preference.)

The American group, however, typically answered based on external cues, such as:

- "I have finished my plate."
- "Others have finished eating."
- "The TV show I'm watching is over."

Is it any surprise that the heavier a person was—American or French—the more they were influenced by external cues as opposed to internal cues to tell them when to stop eating?

It's not too late to start tuning into what's really going on in your body, bringing an inside-out approach to the eating process. By simply bringing this concept into your field of awareness, you're already one step closer to aligning with your inherent wisdom.

Evaluating Hunger Levels

When was the last time you ate until you were so uncomfortably full it hurt? It's interesting that despite the physical, emotional, psychological, and spiritual pain we feel from doing this to ourselves, we do it again and again and again.

Because we've created such strong habits around food that are completely unrelated to physical hunger, how do we teach ourselves to tune into our bodies to know when to start and stop eating? The hunger scale is a tool that can help you. In this practice you turn your attention away from the thinking mind and toward the feeling body. The more you practice, the more your body "speaks" to you and the more you can access your inner wisdom. Practicing present-moment awareness is being still and listening to your body and what it needs; simply check in and listen.

The Hunger Scale

The hunger level scale ranges from 1 to 10, with 1 being the most hungry—the way you feel after you've been sick and not eaten for a few days—and 10 being how full you were at your aunt's house for Christmas last year after you unbuttoned your jeans and went back for a third plate.

The middle point, at 5, is how you feel when you're not hungry or full—you're feeling neutral. You could eat, but you could go without eating as well. This is the point at which a lot of overeating happens because although there's no hunger, there's no fullness either, and we can easily be triggered by something to eat (think: there's always room for _____).

It's best to eat at the 2 to 3 range. If you let yourself get down to a 1 on the scale, you might be setting yourself up to overeat.

Exercise #2: The Hunger Scale in Practice: Beginning, Middle, and End

1. **Check in on hunger level before eating.** Before you start to put food in your mouth, it's best to take a few moments to get grounded and relax (remember, the first REAL step to mindful

eating is *relax*). Next, determine your level of hunger. On the scale from 1 to 10, how hungry are you? Even if you're extremely hungry, a 1 on the scale, give yourself a moment of pause before you eat. If you can do this, you will be able to acknowledge what your hunger level is.

2. **Halfway hunger level check-in.** When you are halfway through your meal, put your eating utensil down, pause, and assess your hunger level once again. On the scale from 1 to 10, are you still hungry (3–4), neutral (5–6), or getting full (7–8)?

3. **End of meal hunger check-in.** After you stop eating, evaluate your level of hunger one last time. Are you feeling comfortably full? Is this a new feeling for you? How does it feel not to overstuff? Was this challenging to do? Are you feeling like you've overeaten? What have you learned through this process?

4. **Journal it.** Write down your experience, using self-compassion, exploring what you learned about yourself that you could carry forward with you into your future meals.

When I go through the hunger level scale in my mindful eating workshops, it's always amazing to hear people describe how often they eat when they're not hungry. The hunger scale is a simple yet remarkably empowering tool to strengthen inner body awareness and guide you through the eating process.

If you find that you're very caught up in your thoughts and can't feel much going on in your body at first, focus on whatever sensations you can feel. This is always a good place to start. Don't be discouraged; if you've been neglecting this awareness for most of your life (as most of us have), it will take time to wake up that inner connection. It's never too late to start; you just need to start where you are.

"If you actually listen to what your body (not your mind) wants, you'll discover that it doesn't want three weeks of hot fudge sundaes..."

—**Geneen Roth,** *Women Food and God*

When to Stop Eating

Even if you're willing to check in with yourself using the hunger scale, how do you actually know when you should stop eating? This is a good question. In Japanese culture there is a saying that goes *"hara hachi bu,"* which means: "eat until you are four-fifths full," or about 80 percent full. It just so happens that the Japanese have the world's highest number of centenarians (one hundred years or older), with research that shows the impact of "under-eating" on longevity.

When incorporating the hunger scale into your mealtime, you can learn to tune into your level of hunger so you become aware of how full you are and give yourself the chance to put the fork down and stop eating. It may also give you the opportunity to look at old, outdated belief systems (BS) you carry about "cleaning your plate" and other BS that no longer serves the new healthy vision of your life.

Exercise #3: Checking In

Once you've evaluated your hunger level, if you notice that you want to eat but you're not actually hungry, explore what's really going on for you. One method you can use to check in with yourself is to ask a few simple questions.

Listed below are ten questions to ask yourself before you eat. You can ask yourself all or just some of the questions that really speak to you. I recommend that you print this out and have it with you for at least the next three days, or post it on your fridge and run through the list before you open the fridge door.

Listen intuitively as your inner wisdom speaks to you:

1. Am I actually experiencing physical hunger? Does my body really want food right now?
2. Am I thirsty instead of hungry? Should I be reaching for water instead of food?
3. Am I using food to suppress, move away from, or avoid feeling an emotion?
4. Am I feeling bored and looking for a distraction or a way to procrastinate?
5. Am I feeling tired? Do I need to sleep instead of eat?

6. Am I feeling pressured to eat due to a social situation? To be polite or because "everyone else is eating?"

7. What kind of hunger am I feeling? Where am I feeling it in my body? Is my soul hungry for deeper meaning and purpose? Is my heart hungry for love? Are my eyes hungry for something visually pleasant? Is this stomach hunger I feel?*

8. What is it that my body truly feels like eating? Is this hunger or a craving?

9. How do I think I will feel after I eat this?

10. Can I eat this without feeling guilty?

As you ask yourself these questions, notice what emotions arise within you. No judgment, just notice. This practice allows you to tune into what you really want or need; then you are in a position to fulfill that desire for yourself. If you are feeling lonely and emotionally hungry, maybe as an alternative you can pick up the phone and call a friend. Are you feeling like you need to show yourself some love? Maybe you can make a cup of tea, light some candles, and take a bath instead of grabbing a bag of chips and hitting the couch. Are you feeling hungry but want to reach for something that you know you'll feel guilty about? Ask yourself what it is that your body really needs to feel nourished.

It's also important to note that if you check in with your hunger level and run through the questions and you discover that you're not actually hungry, it doesn't mean that you "shouldn't" eat or should "restrict" yourself from eating. That's for you to decide. If you would like to receive comfort from food, being conscious of that decision is a great place to start. Most importantly, proceed to eat mindfully and simply pay attention and notice (with a healthy dose of self-compassion) what comes up for you as you offer yourself comfort in this way.

Noticing that you want to eat when you're not hungry is a big step toward self-awareness. There is no need to use this as ammunition against yourself. It would be easy to fall into "I'm not hungry and I want to eat anyway because I'm lonely—*what's*

---

* Refer to Jan Chozen Bays' book *Mindful Eating* for further exploration of the seven kinds of hunger.

wrong with me?" way of thinking. This is where self-compassion comes in. Noticing is a huge first step in the right direction; you should be thrilled that you are able to become aware of this thought. Use this awareness to propel you further on this path, not dig yourself a deeper hole.

A = Awareness

You've probably heard the riddle: if a tree falls in the forest and no one is there to witness it, does it make a sound? What about this riddle: if you eat food but are not mindful of it, do you actually experience and taste it? My answer: *not at all.* In order to reap the many benefits that food has to offer us, awareness needs to be a part of the equation.

What Are You Aware Of?

Once you start to tune into the eating process, you realize there are many things going on while you are eating. There are different layers of reality that you can bring your attention to on the physical, mental, emotional, and spiritual level.

1. **Outer reality**. Awareness of your outer environment and surroundings, including people, or the smell, sight, or sounds of food
2. **Inner reality**. Inner body awareness, emotional awareness, thought awareness, impulse and desire or craving awareness, hunger awareness
3. **Outer reality meets inner reality**. Awareness of actually putting food in your mouth and the sensations that unfold from there; awareness of chewing, taste, flavor, texture, digestion, fullness of stomach
4. **Ultimate reality**. Awareness of the total interconnection between all sentient beings, the connectedness that everything shares, awareness of the miracle of food, awareness of the divine life-force, food as fuel for your life's purpose

There are many mindful eating practices you can use to nurture a positive relationship with food. You can focus your awareness on specific aspects of your inner/outer realities, where these two realities meet or connect, the ultimate reality, or a combination of both.

Exercise #4: Mindful Eating Practice

The following mindful eating practice guides you through various aspects of the four layers of reality. You can do this exercise with a single raisin, cherry, strawberry, or any bite of whole food. My preferred choice is a grape. This practice is a guideline to help you tune into what you are experiencing as you eat, in an open, non-judgmental way.

For this mindful eating exercise, bring yourself back to when you were a child and everything was totally fresh and new. You didn't have names or "labels" for everything yet; the smallest things sparked your curiosity. There was no need to define anything as good or bad. Now, imagine you are looking at this grape for the first time, exploring new territory with total curiosity and no judgment.

With that frame of reference in mind:

1. Pick up this intriguing edible in your hand.
2. Look at it in the palm of your hand. Drink it in with your eyes. The color, the shape, the smoothness, the way it reflects light, the contour.
3. Bring it up to your nose. What does it smell like?
4. Close your eyes and place it between your fingers. What does it feel like? Notice the weight of it in your hand.
5. Bring it to your mouth, noticing the hand-to-mouth motion.
6. Touch it to your lips and notice if you're salivating.
7. Place it in your mouth and notice what it feels like. What does it feel like when it touches the different parts of your mouth?
8. Now take your first bite into this miraculous piece of food. Notice the sound it makes in your mouth.
9. Chew very slowly, but do not swallow it at this point.
10. Notice the sensations of flavors on the various parts of your tongue.
11. Notice any increased salivation.
12. Observe the different textures, and feel the contrast of the inner juiciness with the outer skin.
13. Pay attention to what you're experiencing without any labeling.
14. Notice your impulse to swallow without actually swallowing.
15. When you're ready, swallow.

16. In your mind's eye, follow this hydrating morsel all the way down your esophagus and into your belly. Imagine all the different interactions that are happening with this morsel of food in your body right now. What does that look like and feel like?

17. Take a moment to connect with the energy that is being unlocked as it assimilates into your body.

18. Imagine how your body will use this for energy to enable you to move and to think.

19. Now ask yourself: "What am I spending this precious energy on in my life? How am I using this food to fuel and support my life's purpose?"

20. Allow yourself a moment to sit with this last question and then reflect. What was your experience? How many bites of food would you have typically eaten during this time? What has this experience taught you?

L = Loving-kindness

In my consulting practice, people often tell me they don't know how to love themselves. Whether they are saying it in those exact words or not, that is the message. It seems that in the West, self-criticism and self-denigration are an inherent part of our culture. Our individualistic society helps to foster a mentality of "I'm bad" or "I'm not good enough" that so many people accept as the truth. Stepping onto the mindful path means we become warriors of fierce kindness* toward others and ourselves. We've already touched upon many of the qualities of loving-kindness: honesty, acceptance, compassion, mindfulness, self-care, and feeling good or staying positive when we have insight into our less-than-optimal behavioral patterns. Loving-kindness is unconditional, the way a mother loves her child. As resistant as we may feel toward loving ourselves, we can learn to develop this heartfelt wish in order to be happy and free of suffering.

Maitri: The Practice of Loving-Kindness

There is a story about a monk from the East who came to share the wisdom traditions with a Western audience. After spending time teaching he noticed something

---

* The first time I heard this concept of "fierce kindness" was in Sasha Loring's book *Eating with Fierce Kindness: A Mindful and Compassionate Guide to Losing Weight,* a very handy pocket-sized book.

remarkably different about our culture that he found difficult to comprehend: the level of self-loathing and self-criticism that seemed to be uniquely Western. There is no real concept within the Eastern traditions of not liking oneself. As I studied the wisdom traditions, I learned they have words for concepts that are unknown in the West. The words we use and the meanings that we attach to them are part of what makes up a culture. The wisdom traditions use words to reflect an unconditional love for oneself that we unfortunately lack in the West. But the use of these words in our culture is starting to take root and has become more mainstream. One of these words is *maitri*.

Maitri is a word that comes from the Eastern meditation traditions. This word translates to "loving-kindness" and is used interchangeably with the word *metta*— meaning "friendliness," "gentleness," or "kindness." Maitri is the practice of making friends with ourselves and accepting ourselves exactly as we are in the present moment. Maitri means being a gentle friend towards ourselves when we need kind words and a compassionate heart during difficult times, and is an essential component of self-compassion. When we develop maitri, there is an implied willingness to protect ourselves against the harshness of our own minds and self-critical attitudes.

The ongoing practice of maitri has been a major influence in my life. It has literally altered the way I look at, and interact with, the world. With maitri, you notice your patterns without blame, but rather with an attitude of self-acceptance. This acceptance is by no means passive. It's not about giving up. It's quite the opposite. Maitri is like wrapping yourself in a blanket of loving-kindness that prevents you from spiraling out of control.

Neuroscientists at the University of Wisconsin conducted brain-imaging studies of Buddhist monks (both men and women) meditating on loving-kindness and compassion, and what they discovered was literally mind-altering. The part of the brain associated with empathy and maternal love was more active in the seasoned Buddhist meditators than the control group of non-meditators.[114]

Exercise #5: Practicing Maitri

Although this loving-kindness practice isn't a direct mindful eating practice, learning to foster more self-love and self-respect will indeed influence and benefit your relationship with food. This practice may give you insight into how you may be using food to fill a space in your life that can only be filled with love, one of the most deep-seated reasons so many of us turn to food when we're not hungry.

The practice of maitri often involves the use of phrases. It uses aspirations followed by a heartfelt wish that others enjoy happiness in their lives. The traditional Buddhist practice of maitri uses the aspiration "May all sentient beings enjoy happiness and the root of happiness," but you can put the essence of this aspiration into your own words. Use what feels right for you.

You may choose to use any of the following sentences, or simply come up with your own:

- "May I be safe."
- "May I be healthy."
- "May I be happy."
- "May I have openness of heart."
- "May I live with ease."

The practice of maitri is about connecting to a genuine feeling of loving-kindness that we already have and then gradually foster and strengthen that feeling. This is not about being fake or phony; it's about authentically connecting to where you can feel love and starting from there.

In the traditional practice, you begin with yourself, but for many people this is the most difficult place to start. Personally, I like to start with someone else whom I love, as I find it easier. I invite you to start wherever feels easiest for you.

1. Relax into your body and into your breath. Connect with someone that you love unconditionally; someone you sincerely love. I always start with my mother, because this is the easiest way for me to connect with the feeling of loving-kindness. Experience what it feels like to connect to this feeling, and then send out your wish to that person: *"May you be happy, may you be safe, may you be healthy."* Rest with this feeling as long as you like.

2. Holding the vibration of pure love that you feel for this person, shift this feeling towards yourself. Notice what this feels like. Apply

the aspiration to yourself now: *"May I be happy, may I be safe, may I be healthy."* Rest here as long as is necessary for you.

3. Imagine sending the growing feeling of loving-kindness to a dear friend, repeating the aspiration that feels most appropriate to you.

4. Extend this feeling now to someone about whom you feel neutral or indifferent: perhaps to a person who delivers your mail, or a cashier that you met in passing. Send them the feeling that you've cultivated, along with an aspiration, such as: *"May you be happy, may you be safe, may you be healthy."*

5. Next move to a person you find more challenging or difficult. It may take some time to genuinely send them a heartfelt aspiration. Rest with this feeling and notice what comes up for you.

6. Bring all five people into your awareness and imagine them in a circle around you, radiating light. Extend your aspiration to them. *"May I and (name the five people—my beloved, my friend, my neighbor or neutral person, and the challenging person) all be happy, may we all be safe, may we all be healthy."*

7. Imagine this light extending out to all those around you in your neighborhood, then extending out to all those around you in your city, then your country—moving out bigger and bigger, eventually sending this loving light and aspiration out to everyone in the world. *"May we all be happy, may we all be safe, may we all be healthy."*

After you've finished this exercise, take a few moments to sit quietly and write in your journal. Note any reflections or insights you may have received from this loving-kindness practice.

Bringing Loving-Kindness to the Awareness Process

When you start to incorporate mindfulness into your life, initially it can be difficult to face your ingrained food-related habits. It was very upsetting when I first started to realize how much I had been hurting myself over many years. It's possible that when you come face to face with how you have perpetuated these harmful behaviors, you may feel down and discouraged. Remember that awareness is your starting point in making positive, long-lasting changes to your lifestyle.

The fact that you can acknowledge and see your behavior clearly, even *after* a binge or an overeating episode, is a good thing. This is self-awareness in action. It may be clear in that moment that you are avoiding feeling something, or you recognize that you just want to numb out and use a binge as a way to accomplish that. The fact that you can see the situation clearly is something to celebrate, not something to feel bad about! These insights are your inner wisdom speaking directly to you. This creates the space to say, "I see clearly what I just did. What can I learn from this?" instead of "I can't believe I did this again; I'm a complete failure." To adopt mindfulness means to accept the present moment with compassion, non-judgment, and loving-kindness, and to remember that every single moment is an opportunity to begin anew!

Think of it this way: when you are unable to connect with your inner wisdom and have clear insight about your food patterns, it's as though you're being tossed and turned by waves in a dark, unpleasant pool, unable to see that there's a ladder hanging over you to grab hold of. *Recognizing* that you just went on another binge (or ate mindlessly, or ate unhealthy foods, etc) is like grabbing hold of the first rung of the ladder. Now you can use your past mistakes as an opportunity to learn, to grow, and to deepen your connection with yourself, taking the next step up the ladder. If you can look at your habitual patterns without using them as ammunition to put yourself down ("I'm so terrible; I did it again"), and instead think, "I see now what I did, and this causes me pain. I'm ready to stop doing this to myself." This is the first step up the ladder toward lasting change.

Pulling yourself up on this first rung and out of the pool of suffering takes a tremendous amount of courage, acceptance, and self-love, but it gets easier. Focus on stepping up one rung at a time. It may be a slow, lifelong climb, but trust and remember that climbing up is better than the alternative. As the wisdom traditions teach, when you begin to see what causes your suffering, you start to recognize the suffering of others and realize that this is our shared humanity. You can begin to soften your heart and have compassion for yourself and others, and set the aspiration that we can all ease our suffering and connect to happiness, contentment, and peace.

Off the Hook

Try to commit to one mindful meal at least every other day, and as you gradually become more fluent in the REAL Food Approach to Mindful Eating, start applying mindfulness in a wider range of situations: while grocery shopping, while preparing meals, and at restaurants. Put in that extra little effort to eat in a nice, relaxing,

PART FIVE

The Emotional Hook

"One can overcome the forces of negative emotions, like anger and hatred, by cultivating their counter-forces, like love and compassion."

—Dalai Lama

Chapter 9

How Our Emotions Hook Us

At one point in my life, *Confessions of an Emotional Eater* could have been the title of my autobiography. I used food as a coping mechanism to distract, avoid, procrastinate, numb out, tune out, and check out. Food was my security blanket and I constantly used it to alter my moods in some way or another. I used it for emotional support, to suppress, comfort, or avoid feelings of sadness, loneliness, boredom, worry, and even excitement. I could go on, but I'll spare you the excessive details. More importantly, do *you* recognize yourself in any of these statements?

Everyone uses food in diverse ways to serve different purposes in their lives. We all create strong emotional ties to food; sometimes we're conscious of this, but most of the time we're not. We are emotional beings by nature, and our emotions are one of the main reasons we're triggered to overeat. According to Jane Jakubczak, Registered Dietitian and Coordinator of Nutrition Services at the University of Maryland, 75 percent of overeating is caused by emotions.[115] This makes addressing emotional eating and learning how to deal with emotions of prime importance.

Being emotional is nothing to be ashamed of—our emotions are a blessing, albeit sometimes in disguise. They are like the signposts to our inner world. Emotions provide us with useful information about how we are doing or how we are coping at any given point in time, and they guide our behavior. Mindless emotional eating is a clear indication that something is out of balance in our lives, and if we are willing to listen, we can take it as a sign that we have some inner work to do.

The Whys of Emotional Eating

Eating is an emotional experience and involves emotions from the present and past. There are many subconscious factors involved in our emotional relationship with food; these factors are what determine how much we eat, when we eat, and for what reasons we eat. They may include the internal dialogue or the stories we tell ourselves about our relationship with food, including our history with food and our experience with food as children, how much self-awareness we have around food, how worthy we feel we are, how we learn to cope with stress, and how we learn to process intense emotions. All of these aspects can and do play a role in our emotional relationship with food.

In the remaining part of this chapter we will explore three important questions that will help you to better understand emotional eating:

1. Why do we tend to turn away from, instead of face, our emotions?
2. Why do we tend to turn to food instead of processing our emotions on a physical, energetic level?
3. How do different types of foods affect us emotionally?

Learning to Stay with Unpleasant Emotions

Most emotional eaters can acknowledge that they use food to avoid emotions they don't want to feel. Eating then becomes a form of distraction. *Shenpa* is a Tibetan word popularized by author and spiritual teacher Pema Chödrön* that helps to shed light on this tendency to distract ourselves with food. A simple translation of *shenpa* points to "attachment," but Pema Chödrön offers another word—"hooked." *Shenpa* is about how we get hooked. Other words that point to the underlying essence of *shenpa* are "urge" or "triggered." Sound familiar?

Shenpa is not easy to describe, but I assure you it's something that everyone has experienced. It's about how we, as human beings, habitually get triggered by

---

* To further explore Pema Chödrön's teachings on *shenpa*, please refer to her audio course *Getting Unstuck: Breaking Your Habitual Patterns and Encountering Naked Reality*, produced by Sounds True, or read one of her many incredible books, including *Taking the Leap: Freeing Ourselves from Old Habits and Fears*, published by Shambhala.

something (it could be anything), and almost instantaneously we automatically close down to ourselves and to others. We then get stuck in a place of "unpleasant feeling" and then immediately look for ways to move away from the present moment to avoid feeling what we're feeling.

Pema recounts a helpful analogy passed on to her by Dzigar Kongtrul Rinpoche to help explain *shenpa*. She says we are all like little children with a bad case of poison ivy. We know that if we scratch it, we will experience some immediate relief, a temporary moment of satisfaction, but because we're just children, we don't know that when we scratch it—when we give into the underlying urge to scratch—we end up making matters worse. We get hooked on scratching, and despite making us feel better initially, it ultimately causes suffering. Before we know it, we're scratching and scratching and all we feel is pain. We become totally consumed by the itch and the need to scratch it, and it takes over every single aspect of our lives. We can't stop thinking about it, and eventually it gets out of control and the end result is suffering. The first time I heard this story, I felt like I was struck by lightning. I knew this was the perfect metaphor for my relationship with food and my underlying struggle.

There are many ways we can experience *shenpa*, what Pema describes as that familiar urge to "scratch." You're speaking with your partner, and all of sudden he or she says something to you that you feel is hurtful, and you have an immediate reaction. You go from being emotionally open to instantly shutting down. It can almost feel beyond your control, much in the same way you may experience the "fight or flight" stress response as an involuntary reaction. It's a protective response, and in that instant, you do anything to avoid, deny, and escape what you're feeling in the present moment. You may find yourself swept away by the tidal wave of reactionary thoughts and story lines about why they are wrong, you are right, you are the victim, they are the perpetrators, and so on. Or you find yourself engaging in your knee-jerk reactive behavioral patterns in whatever way that looks like for you: picking up the remote, grabbing a beer, surfing the web, or standing in front of the refrigerator picking at last night's leftovers.

Whether we feel a sense of insecurity, fear, or just a general uneasiness, the immediate reaction is to push away what we don't want to feel and immediately find something to replace it with. We tend to do this by seeking pleasure or comfort or by numbing out, all of which can be accomplished through eating. The more we give into the urge, the more we scratch it, the less ability we develop to simply *stay* with what is arising for us in the moment, creating strong habitual patterns of avoidance and seeking out pleasure. This is how cravings can have such a strong hold on us. We equate the food of our desire with relief from suffering.

"The sad part is that all we're trying to do is not feel that underlying uneasiness. The sadder part is that we proceed in such a way that the uneasiness only gets worse. The message here is that the only way to ease our pain is to experience it fully. Learn to stay. Learn to stay with uneasiness, learn to stay with tightening, learn to stay with the itch and urge of shenpa, so that the habitual chain reaction doesn't continue to rule our lives, and the patterns that we consider unhelpful don't keep getting stronger as the days and months and years go by."

—**Pema Chödrön,** *Taking the Leap*

Scratching the Itch

Everyone has a tendency to seek temporary comfort in things that ultimately hurt them, the way that scratching the itch ultimately brings more pain. Food just happens to be one of the sources of so-called "comfort"—others include sex, alcohol, drug use, smoking, checking e-mails, getting angry, overworking, shopping, or watching TV. Instead of allowing ourselves to feel, we often resort to any number of these things to numb our feelings or distract ourselves with pleasure.

After much pain and suffering has been endured, we may eventually realize that we have a choice: we can develop courage, strength, and loving-kindness toward ourselves and directly experience the underlying itch without scratching (recognizing a craving and not acting on it), or we can continue to scratch and bleed, causing ourselves more pain (returning time after time to eating foods that ultimately make us feel horrible). We can then start to recognize that turning to food yet again, in the same old habitual ways, is actually hurting us more than it's helping us.

There's nothing wrong with wanting or needing comfort. In and of itself, craving is neither good nor bad. Craving becomes a problem when we become attached to "I *need* that; I *want* that; *that* (fill in the blank) will satisfy me and help ease my underlying discomfort or suffering." There's also nothing inherently wrong with turning to food for comfort—if you're eating with mindful awareness and without any guilt, blame, or shame. The real challenge is to ask yourself if turning to food is actually helping you or hurting you. Are you being realistic about what satisfying your craving is really doing for you? As one of my clients said, "It doesn't matter how much chocolate I binge on at night, I still have to wake up in the morning and face my shitty boss." Food can't solve your problems for you. Instead, it usually covers over the original problem and in turn creates an additional food-related problem to focus on.

Energy Drain on the Body

We all process the experiences of our lives differently. Two people can go through a similar challenging situation and choose to handle it very differently. Take grieving, for example. Death is a part of life, and so grieving the loss of a loved one is something that everyone will face. I don't claim to be an expert on the grieving process, but I have seen two main scenarios play out on opposite ends of the spectrum.

Mary is fifty-four; she's grieving the loss of her husband. I met her about six months into her grieving process. She describes herself as extremely emotional, and she's barely able to "stomach" eating. When she weighs herself she is surprised to find that she has lost about fifteen pounds over this period. I see her months later. She states she is less emotional and is eating again, looking healthier and stronger than when I first saw her.

On the other end of the spectrum, my friend Monica has lost one of her really close friends. In conversations with her she does not want to even broach the subject with me. Monica has, by her own admission, been overeating, and she's starting to feel the consequences of excess weight gain: less movement and motivation, low moods, and depressed feelings.

Isn't it interesting how some people process intense emotions and don't really want or ask for food, and others avoid processing their emotions and turn to eating as a way to cope? What's going on here? When we are feeling emotional and turn to food instead of processing what we're feeling, we literally divert energy away from the emotional process and toward digestion. Once you understand why, the reason emotional eaters turn to food as a means of coping starts to make sense.

Vital Nerve Energy

There are many different uses of the word "energy" when it comes to our health. We often refer to energy as "wanting more energy" or "feeling low on energy" and even "feeling the energy in your body."

When we "want more energy" as an antidote to feeling tired, what's being referred to here is a type of electrical energy that is actually a low-voltage electrical current.[116] This electrical energy is also called *vital nerve energy* or *nerve force*, and it is often referred to as "thriving" or "vitality."

Think of the nervous system as a giant telephone network with the brain acting as the main operator. Now imagine that this operating system is run on a large battery, and there's only so much available nerve energy (battery) available at any given time. This battery is constantly being used up with the countless back and forth communication between the brain and the body that result in thoughts, movements, digestion, etc. Every cell in your body requires a continual supply of vital nerve energy from your nervous system.

There are four primary processes that require vital nerve energy:

- **Physiological**: the processes and functions of the body that include repairing and restoring cells, cleansing and detoxifying, digesting food, etc.
- **Physical**: activities that involve movement, like walking, talking, running, playing, taking a shower, mowing the lawn, and cleaning the house.
- **Mental**: thinking and brain processes, such as studying for an exam, working on a puzzle, analyzing a situation, making decisions.
- **Emotional**: thoughts that influence our feelings and feed into emotional reactions, such as stress, anxiety, excitement, excessive worrying, and depression.

Of all these processes, there are two that require a very large amount of vital nerve energy (battery supply): digesting food and processing emotions. Many people believe that food gives us energy. If that is the case, why do people literally pass out right after eating way beyond feeling full? If food provides us with energy, shouldn't we have more energy after eating a huge meal? As it turns out, food is more like fuel, and the processing of this fuel (digestion) requires a lot of battery power (vital nerve energy).

Vital nerve energy is like the battery in your car and the food you eat like the fuel you put in the gas tank.[117] The car will not run without adequate battery supply or fuel supply; both are essential, but they are different. The car won't start without enough battery charge, and the way it runs will depend on the quality of the fuel you put in it. Think of overeating as pouring too much gasoline into the tank and continuing to pour it in after the tank is full, spilling it out all over the ground!

With this information we can see that one way to avoid processing emotions— to avoid feeling what we're feeling—is to mindlessly overeat, directing our energy toward digesting food instead of emoting. Combine this with the types of foods people usually turn to for emotional comfort (highly processed foods filled with sugar, fat, and salt), and what you develop is a very strong and reinforcing habit. The good news is that you can take this information and immediately put it to use, making simple and effective changes that can drastically change your energy levels.

Can you guess the number-one way to recharge your "batteries?" Sleep! This information should empower you to perhaps take a nap instead of scavenge for hyper-palatable foods when you're tired. It's also worth making an effort to steer clear of all stimulants such as caffeine when you're looking for an energy boost, as these are a major drain on vital nerve energy. Can you guess what kind of fuel is best for your engine? You probably guessed it: real, whole foods, specifically fruits and vegetables. Eating these foods requires the least amounts of digestive energy, so to speak, and therefore frees up your energy to focus on other important things in life, such as dealing with your emotional needs directly, so you can in turn thrive and *live your joyful life's purpose.*

Cues and Attachment of Meaning

When we looked at why we overeat from an environmental and physical perspective (in both Parts One and Two), we discussed how "cues" can trigger us to eat, overeat, or eat when we're not hungry. One of the reasons that cues trigger us is because we attach meaning—*on an emotional level*—to these cues. Again, from an evolutionary perspective, this was and is essential to our species' survival.

> **"But much of survival learning is based on internal reward systems that have evolved along with the emotional limbic brain. These reward systems are based on the brain's neurotransmitters, chemicals that promote message transfer from neuron to neuron. And not surprisingly, most of the neurotransmitters that provide reward are primarily within the emotional brain and its connections."**
>
> **—Robert Scaer,** *8 Keys to Brain-Body Balance*

As a biological imperative, we are driven to attach emotional meaning to things, events, and people and quickly incorporate new information into our already-existing cognitive database. We either like or dislike something, some place, or someone; we make positive or negative associations; we tend to crave or avoid; we experience comfort or discomfort. This built-in mechanism is very useful in many instances, hence the expression, "once burned, twice shy." We burn ourselves once, and we label that as painful and associate it to a feeling of discomfort, and now the visual cue of a red-hot burner reminds us *without us needing to think about it* that this is hot and will hurt if we touch it again.

The same applies to food. Cues that are associated with the pleasure response are learned and "locked in" to emotional memory very quickly. We feel emotional distress, we turn to food (and all it takes is once), and we quickly feel better because it releases feel-good brain chemicals like dopamine and serotonin. This is one of the ways that emotional eating can lead to an addiction to hyper-palatable foods: because these foods evoke a "hyper-pleasurable" response in us, we keep going back for more. When we understand overeating from this perspective, it is clear that whenever we are feeling low or any kind of emotional distress, we immediately return to the foods that give us the *most* reward or pleasurable feelings.

This hyper-pleasurable response gets locked into your *memories*, and the next time you feel this emotional distress, you remember that you felt better by eating these foods—even if you are not conscious of it. You equate the food consumed during an emotional eating episode (usually an *over*eating episode) to the primary response of a positive, pleasurable feeling (comfort), despite a longer and negative secondary response of "low" feeling that follows overeating. So despite the fact that twenty minutes after you eat the whole darn tub of ice cream you feel terrible, what your brain remembers is that initial good-feeling response. And now that we know the foods that give us the most intense pleasurable response are processed foods high in sugar, fat, and salt (even some "health" foods fall into this category), we have one more reason to steer clear of them, focus on emotional stability, and improve our relationship with food.

Cortisol, Serotonin, and Food Addiction

Although many people struggle with food, overeating, and weight, it's obviously not a problem for everyone. What makes some people susceptible to food addiction while others are not? Research shows that people susceptible to alcohol and food addiction may have a malfunction in serotonin production.[118] Serotonin is a neurotransmitter in the brain that promotes peacefulness and relaxation, decreases anxiety, and provides relief from pain. Serotonin also is depleted by chronic stress. So on top of some people's inability (by no fault of their own) to produce this very important "feel-good" chemical, they're also dealing with serotonin depletion from the everyday stresses of life.

When we lead fulfilling lives—we do the work we love, we have close friends and a solid social network, we make time for physical activity and cope with stress effectively—we're not likely to turn to food for support, because all these activities give us our daily dose of happy brain chemicals that we need to feel good and emotionally balanced.

Everyone goes through tough times—it's part of life. But it's how we relate to and perceive difficult situations that really make the difference. If we trust the process of life with a "this too shall pass" attitude, with a knowing that things will turn around, then we may experience times of lower levels of feel-good brain chemicals but allow space for ourselves to simply "be where we are." However, when we feel like there's no end in sight, and feelings of loneliness, sadness, anger, or alienation seem all consuming, we're more likely to turn to something to help supplement our much-needed feel-good brain chemicals. And it's quite understandable that we'd turn to the most readily available, cheap, and legal "hit" we can get—hyper-palatable food—because we've already experienced the pleasure these foods can offer us and have thus already habituated to them.

It then becomes understandable why people with a chemical deficiency of serotonin may turn to refined sugar for the "extra support," as sugar has a powerful effect on serotonin levels in the brain.[119] When we consume refined carbohydrates, serotonin is manufactured and released in the brain, providing quick and temporary relief from stress or pain. Even with a temporary fix, the brain will quickly store this information into our memories—and what we have just acquired is a coping mechanism rooted in a very powerful biological process. This may explain why many millions of Americans have subconsciously developed an emotional dependence to food.

As discussed in chapter 3, dopamine is not only released when we eat but also before we eat, to help us focus our attention and *motivate* our behavior toward obtaining the food of our desire. This also has an effect on cortisol—one of the main stress hormones. Cortisol is released to kick our butts into gear, lending us motivation to pursue the food. But remember that stress also triggers our automatic mind (responsible for activating deeply rooted habits) at the expense of our conscious mind. Future thoughts of fitting into our slim jeans go out the window, and we focus on immediate gratification. Stress also inhibits the neuroplasticity, making it more difficult to adopt new healthier habits.

Pause & Reflect: Eating Your Emotions

Consider the following statements, by answering yes or no. Your responses may help you explore and uncover emotional eating tendencies.

Do I tend to:

1. Eat more when I'm stressed out or nervous?
2. Eat more when I'm feeling lonely?
3. Eat more if I'm angry or upset?
4. Overeat more when I'm alone rather than in the company of others?
5. Eat when I'm in a great mood because eating makes me feel even better
6. Eat to celebrate good news?
7. Turn to food when I hear disappointing news?
8. Use food to calm down worried thoughts?
9. "Tune out" when I'm overeating and feel guilt or shame afterwards?
10. Eat when I feel bored?

Fueling the Fire: How the Cycle Continues

We've all turned to something for comfort and support that in turn makes us feel worse. I know what it's like to be there—waking up from a binge is never a pretty picture. It doesn't make sense, but we all do it to some degree and in our own ways. Why do we do it? All the things most of us repeatedly reach for are just attempts to feel better—and who really wants to feel bad? Consider it a kind gesture from your unconscious self to help you reach for those familiar good feelings that we all inherently long for.

So the cycle continues: we feel bad, reaching for foods to make us feel better; we feel better for a moment, realize that we did it again, feel bad again, and know exactly what will make us feel better—but alas, only temporarily. In this way we look for strength and comfort in what ultimately hurts, disempowers, and weakens us.

Because food has such a strong influence on our emotions, and our emotions in turn influence what we choose to eat, self-reinforcing patterns emerge. Since these patterns tend to perpetuate themselves, we lose sight of the original cause of the emotional distress.

Getting Unhooked

When eating becomes your main strategy for managing emotions, you will invariably deal with the consequences. The obvious consequences are physical, but when you repeatedly turn to food to fill a void that has nothing to do with physical hunger, the results can only be disappointing. As the song goes, it's like "looking for love in all the wrong places."

Your desire for hyper-palatable foods when you're sad, upset, tired, lonely, frustrated, excited, and angry is not a moral weakness or lack of willpower. If you've repeatedly turned to food to manage your emotions, with an inner knowing that you are ultimately making matters worse, you may have also entered the seemingly endless cycle of self-criticism. Millions of people also fall into this same cycle every single day. These foods evoke powerful responses in us—*so stop feeling bad about it already!* You are not morally weak or a failure; you're like the millions of others who genuinely want to lead a happy and fulfilled life and just need a little guidance to get there!

The next chapter can empower you to take a completely new direction in life, one that doesn't involve dependence on these drug-like foods for emotional support. Instead you can learn how to cope and work with your emotions in effective ways, reduce your dependence on food as a coping mechanism, and establish a healthy, balanced relationship with real, whole food.

Chapter 10

Unhooked: Working with Emotions and Boosting the Feel-Good Chemicals in Your Brain Naturally

I f you want to heal emotional eating, you have to address and work with your emotions directly. Most of us have never had such training. Actually we learned to do quite the opposite—to distract, to avoid, and (for many of you reading this book) to stuff your emotions down with food.

When you shift to eating real, whole foods, you may experience physical detoxification (headaches, nausea, tiredness, flu-like symptoms), as well as a variety of emotional states. As discussed in chapter 9, the more you free up your digestive capacity, the more energy you have to address and process emotions directly.

One of the best ways to work with emotional eating is to stabilize and balance your emotions. In addition to eating a whole foods diet and practicing self-compassion, you can boost the natural feel-good chemicals in your brain through incorporating meditation and exercise into your daily routine, as well as getting better quality sleep.

Boost #1: Incorporate Mindfulness Meditation into Your Day

Don't be frightened or put off by the word—meditation is just a general term used for any practice that involves training the mind to become more present and aware. Although meditation is an Eastern practice, you certainly don't have to be a yogi or a Buddhist to reap the many benefits of meditation. Meditation has become mainstream in our Western culture with classes, retreats, workshops, how-to meditate books, and online courses. It's a secular practice; anyone from any faith can learn meditation.

There are many different kinds of meditation: sitting, kneeling, walking, eating, or standing; meditations that teach us how to let go of thoughts or to focus on an object, or concentrate on creating awareness of the senses. Any form of prayer or mantra repetition can also be considered a meditation. There are also visualization mediations, as well as the well-known transcendental meditation (TM) that many celebrities like Paul McCartney and Oprah Winfrey openly endorse—and for good reason.

The Many Benefits of Meditation Practice

Remember that we have one brain but two minds: the automatic mind and the conscious mind. Meditation is a central practice in strengthening the conscious mind, the mind that helps us commit to and follow through on our goals. Even if you only commit anywhere from five to twenty minutes a day, meditation is shown to improve a wide range of self-control skills and has many other benefits, including:[120]

- Increased focus and attention (including ignoring distractions)
- Improved memory and other cognitive processes like problem solving
- Stress management
- Reduces fatigue and anxiety
- Reduces mood disturbances (stabilizes mood)
- Promotes psychological well-being
- Helps with impulse control
- Improves self-awareness
- Improves emotional resiliency
- Increased efficiency of our autonomic nervous system

The reason we experience these benefits is because our brain is like a muscle that we can train and work out. Just as our muscles receive an increased blood flow when we lift weights, blood flow also increases to the prefrontal cortex (PFC) when we meditate. This leads to increased gray matter and neural connections in the PFC and other areas of the brain related to self-awareness. In one study, researchers detected increased gray matter volume in regions of the meditator's mind associated with emotional regulation and response control. The authors of the study go on to say, "Thus, larger volumes in these regions might account for meditators' singular abilities and habits to cultivate positive emotions, retain emotional stability, and engage in mindful behavior."[121]

Based on the positive impact that mindfulness has on our physical health and mental well-being, it's no surprise that researchers are now exploring the benefits of mindfulness for people with a range of disordered eating. One mindfulness intervention training program called MB-EAT, developed by Jean Kristeller, is shown to help decrease binge-eating episodes, improve one's sense of self-control with regard to eating, and diminish depressive symptoms.[122]

Mindfulness meditation can be used to help curb cravings and prevent food addiction relapse. This makes the simple practice of meditation worth its weight in gold. It also makes meditation one of your most readily available, easily accessible tools at your disposal to help unhook you from your food-related struggle. You can use meditation as a replacement for the feel-good hit you've been getting from hyper-palatable food, as regular meditation is shown to release dopamine in the brain, helping you to feel good naturally.[123]

Impermanence and Emotional Discomfort

Everyone knows that life is unpredictable. Impermanence and constant change are the only things of which we can be certain. Even though we may be able to acknowledge this on an intellectual level, this is a challenging reality for us to grasp emotionally and is often the root cause of our emotional distress. As a result we spend much of our time trying to make life as predictable and permanent as possible. We mistakenly seek comfort by trying to make our life experience solid and concrete; what we are seeking is psychological security. Pema Chödrön describes this as our desire to have "solid ground" under our feet as a way to feel secure in this continuously changing world. We seek this solid ground in many ways: through the perceived solidity and security of a house, a job, relationships, past memories, or plans for the future; we don't want to stay with the ever-changing present moment or "groundlessness," which is the true reality of our existence.

Sitting meditation practice can help us to see the true nature of reality, and accept that everything is always changing and is impermanent. Our thoughts come and go, our breath goes in and out, our emotions and underlying energies come and then dissipate. That's why walking this path takes courage, because we start to uncover and face what we often try to cover up and avoid, and we start to see how often we distract ourselves. Meditation is called a practice for a reason; it takes time to learn to sit with our emotions and to train ourselves to continuously keep coming back to what we feel, over and over again.

Learning to Stay with Discomfort

Meditation practice is about learning to stay present. Committing to this practice, we learn to sit with the underlying discomfort that is inherent in the human condition, despite our extremely low tolerance for discomfort. We've become accustomed to trying to cover over that uneasiness, so we do what we can to move away from it, often seeking comfort in things that ultimately cause us more pain and suffering.

It is difficult to process uncomfortable experiences by pushing away, resisting, or trying to escape. This may sound like bad news. You may be thinking, "I have to actually move *closer* to what I don't want to feel? How will that help me?"

If you are always distracting yourself to avoid feeling emotions, you're never really addressing the core, underlying root of the issue. Ask yourself if the years of avoiding your emotions actually helped you, or caused you more pain? Are you ready for a new solution, one that is rooted in thousands of years of practice and wisdom?

Removing Blocks to Meditation

Misconceptions about meditation create obstacles that prevent people from trying it. One of the basic misconceptions is that when you sit down in your seat in a relaxed position with poise and grace, a calm sense of serenity and tranquility will flush over you. You may benefit from letting go of your preconceived notions of meditation and simply view this as a practice of mindful awareness.

By practicing *mindfulness-awareness* meditation, we connect to and strengthen the mindful quality that is present in everything we do, our inherent capacity to be present, and to simply relax with who we are. This practice is not about transcending or leaving this reality (although some forms of meditation do focus on transcendence) but about firmly rooting ourselves into the present moment, becoming completely awake to the reality of "now."

Meditation is also not about "getting rid" of thoughts. If we try to empty our minds and get rid of our thoughts, what we are doing is actively engaging in a struggle to "clear our heads." Yes, sometimes we experience vast, open spaciousness in our minds, but more often than not, when we first start to meditate, we become acquainted with "busy" mind, also known as "monkey mind." Not only is that perfectly okay, in fact it's quite normal.

The magic of meditation is that gradually, over time, we begin to see the transient quality of our thoughts, and we see that they are not as solid as we thought they were (a good example of groundlessness). With this practice we loosen the grip that our thoughts have over us, and we begin to just relax, deeply relax, with our own minds and learn to be at home with ourselves. We begin to see the transparency or illusion of "busy" mind, and over time we learn to not take it so seriously and eventually make friends with it.

If you want to sit in meditation because you have the desire to move away from feeling bad and only want to cling to feeling good, then you are inevitably setting yourself up for more suffering. Meditation is about feeling whatever it is you feel. It is a complete acceptance of whatever arises with an attitude of gentleness, patience, acceptance, and loving-kindness. It is only when you truly relax with yourself and who you are and what you feel, without grasping at or pushing away any thought or feeling, that you start to see the transformative process of meditation.

Please refer to Appendix C for guidance on basic mindfulness-awareness meditation practice.

Meditation—A Tool for Working with Emotions

Meditation practice is especially useful when working with emotional processes. The practice of working with difficult emotions is to contact the underlying energy of it, and connecting to the physical sensations of what you're feeling in your body. With meditation, you learn to stay with the difficult emotion without trying to alter it, and move towards experiencing it directly while maintaining curiosity about what is going on in the body. As a result of this practice, your difficult emotions will soften over time and loosen their grip on you.

Emotions escalate because we feed their momentum with the stories that are connected to the emotion. We may perpetuate a story that "they" did this to "us," and we were wronged—or whatever the situation may be. This constant internal dialogue keeps us hooked and fuels an emotional reaction. What would happen if we learned to let go of the story line and instead focused our attention on tuning into the underlying sensation of what it is we are truly feeling? When we let the story line go, what we may discover is the underlying physical sensations that we thought were so fixed and solid are actually quite fluid, transient, and always changing. Over time, with practice, when we're feeling intense emotions, this may allow us to loosen our grip of the story line, and possibly even learn how to get better at dropping the story line altogether. When we really go into and surrender to what we're feeling, we can experience the fluidity of our emotions directly. What tends to happen is that they dissipate, or at least slowly de-escalate.

Exercise #1: Surfing the Urge

The next time you notice yourself struggling with an intense emotion or any kind of craving, try this simple technique called "surfing the urge."

Try to move "out of your head" and "into your body." Notice that this craving or emotional energy is like a wave, and instead of being swept away by it, visualize yourself riding out the wave.

Connect to what you are physically feeling. The emotional sensations you feel can be quite intense; it can be hot, cold, pulsating, aching, trembling, constricting, suffocating, expanding, etc. Explore all the sensations that arise with openness, curiosity, and a non-judgmental attitude. What's happening in your body? What does this urge physically feel like? Do you notice any changes in your heart rate, in your body temperature, in your stomach?

At first, I recommend that you practice sitting meditation at more "neutral" times—times when you're not working with intense cravings or emotions, as this can be extremely overwhelming without a solid foundation of practice and/or guidance. Ideally, you are working on flexing your mindfulness muscle to gain enough strength, courage, and loving-kindness for yourself to sit in the midst of a more emotionally intense experience. As you practice, you gradually learn to catch the emotional reaction, sit with it, and drop the story line that's fueling it. Then you feel the bodily sensations totally and completely. This is one way that we learn how to process and deal directly with emotions.

Boost #2: Have More Fun: Exercise and Music

I often tell people that walking saved my life. Walking seems to have this magical power to completely shift a mood, shut down a craving, radically change a negative outlook, and help cope with intense emotions. One of the reasons exercise feels so good is because it can activate the same pleasure pathways as morphine.[124] Exercise is a great, *natural* way to feel good immediately and has been shown to help addicts reduce cravings because it can activate many neurotransmitter systems involved in the addiction process. Physical activity also enhances cognitive and brain function, improves learning and memory, and protects against the development of neurodegenerative diseases.[125]

Exercise and physical activity:

- Decrease stress hormones
- Boost endorphin levels
- Strengthen the immune system
- Improve blood flow and oxygen to the brain
- Reduce physiological reactivity toward stress
- Improve mental health
- Improve emotional and mood stability
- Help with weight management

When choosing a physical activity, it's important to engage in something you love to do. Don't worry about jumping into intense exercise; it's actually better if you start off slowly and gradually increase your strength and stamina in order to avoid putting stress on your system, which may cause you to seek out food for comfort! If you're not enjoying one form of exercise, find another. Walking is a great place to start, because all it requires is a pair of shoes and it's not intimidating in the least. This is an easy first goal to set. I love to use walking as a way not only to get my endorphins flowing, but to let go of or reflect on a difficult situation, decompress from a long day of work, kick start my day with more energy, spend time with a friend, or listen to an audio book on my iPod. Walking is also my favorite way to spend time in nature and commune with the local environment around me.

Music is also a huge pick-me-up and can give you an instant dose of your natural feel-good brain chemicals. One study by researchers at McGill University showed that people experience pleasure in response to music, leading to dopamine release in the brain.[126] This is how we learn to replace unhealthy and addictive "hits" from hyper-palatable food with healthy "hits" like walking, dancing, or listening to music.

If I'm in a rut, feeling down, stressed, or overly emotional, and I can't quite muster up the motivation to get outside and go for a walk (even though I know it would do me a world of good), all I have to do is put on one of my favorite songs, and it immediately evokes a shift in me. Music works like a charm every time. How about a double whammy effect? Combine physical activity with music, also known as dancing! You don't even need to go anywhere; you can put on some great music and dance in your living room. Your neighbors might think you're wacky, but at least you'll feel amazing!

The key is, if you love to do it, and it involves movement, then go for it! Don't think of exercising as laborious; think of it as playful. Find a game to play, team up with someone else and work out with them, play with your kids, get active in your yard or garden, go swimming with the family, or join a hiking group. Do whatever you love to do, preferably outside in nature.

Caution: Rewarding Yourself for Working Out

It is not uncommon for people to notice weight gain rather than weight loss when they start to "work out." There are a couple of different reasons for this. People tend to underestimate the caloric value of food consumed, as well as calories burned through activity. After exercising you may feel like you "deserve a reward," so you overcompensate by eating more than you actually need. Don't fall into this trap!

You can avoid this trap by doing physical activity that you love and that doesn't feel like hard work or punishment. In one study,[127] two groups of people were told they would do a one-mile walk before dinner. Although the walks were identical—same distance, same pace, same time—one group was told the walk was an "exercise walk" and the other group a "scenic walk." When the participants came to dinner after their walk, the researchers measured what individuals in each group consumed. Can you guess the results? The people who were told they were on an exercise walk ate more than the people on the scenic walk, consuming significantly more calories, largely from dessert, suggesting that people were rewarding themselves for their exercise.

Boost #3: Get More and Better Quality Sleep

When I'm tired, I not only become more emotionally reactive, but I notice that one of my primary triggers for making less-than-optimal food choices is lack of sleep. An estimated 50 to 70 million Americans suffer from a chronic sleep and wakefulness disorder, hindering daily functioning and adversely affecting health and longevity.[128] And as it turns out, sleep deprivation makes it more difficult to get a grip on our emotions. The results of one study showed that a sleep-deprived group had a much bigger reaction to emotionally charged images than the other group that had normal levels of sleep.[129] According to Matthew Walker, director of UC Berkeley's Sleep and Neuroimaging Laboratory, "It's almost as though, without sleep, the brain had reverted back to more primitive patterns of activity, in that it was unable to put emotional experiences into context and produce controlled, appropriate responses."[130] This is why when we're tired the littlest nudge can send us off the deep end, and we all know what we tend to want to do when we're feeling emotional—*sit in meditation, right?* Well, at least that's what we're aiming for!

Sleep deprivation also impairs glucose utilization in the body and brain.[131] This means that your cells are not getting the fuel they need, especially the brain cells in your constantly hungry prefrontal cortex, which is responsible for keeping your goals at the forefront of you mind. As a result, sleep deprivation can trigger you to crave glucose—aka sugar. But instead of turning to the beneficial, natural sugars found in whole fruits, most people tend to go for the most widely available form of this quick fix: refined, hyper-palatable packaged foods full of white sugar and its best friends, fat and salt. At the same time, your higher-order decision-making capabilities, like the ability to remember the importance of your long-term goals, get pushed aside as you beeline toward the cookie box.

Sleep deprivation may provoke hormonal changes in the body that impact appetite regulation and increase the chance of overconsuming calories, leading to weight gain. Studies show that sleeping fewer than seven hours per night is linked to a higher Body Mass Index (BMI).[132] If you're sleep deprived and carrying excess weight that you're trying to lose, you're fighting an uphill battle. One study reported that sleep-deprived people ate more than five hundred extra calories a day.[133] That's almost an extra five pounds per month! This is because people are turning to food to wake themselves up because most people believe it will "give them energy" as discussed in the last chapter. But this proves to be an ineffective coping mechanism that actually drains energy further. Lack of sleep increases ghrelin, a hunger-stimulating hormone, and decreases leptin, the hormone that gives us the signal to stop eating due to satiation.[134] Lack of sleep is also shown to decreases insulin sensitivity,[135] correlated with weight gain and diabetes.

Sleep is the only thing that can recharge our batteries (and our goals), and lucky for us—it's free! Good quality sleep is so satisfying and refreshing; who wouldn't want to sleep an extra hour each morning? You may have a million reasons why you can't get more sleep, and maybe some are more important or valid than others, but ultimately it's your health and your choice; isn't it worth making an effort?

Giving up stimulants is one way you can ensure better quality sleep. Many people hold the mistaken belief that stimulants provide energy, when in fact they drastically reduce the long-term energy supply of the body. If you're using any kind of stimulant to "give you energy," including coffee, chocolate, or amphetamines, there's a good chance you may be running dangerously low on energy reserves, eventually leading to what is commonly known as burnout.

How Much Sleep Is Enough?

How do you know if you're sleep deprived? Here are a few key signs:

- You require an alarm clock to wake up every morning
- You notice increased snacking throughout the day (and not because you're exercising more or skipped a meal)
- You crave high-fat, refined, calorie-dense foods
- You feel emotionally reactive, irritable, and moody
- You have difficulty focusing or concentrating, frequent forgetfulness
- You have a weakened immune system and are sick often
- You notice reduced fine motor skills, clumsiness, and dulled reflexes
- You have a decreased sex drive
- You feel a general sense of reduced ambition, drive, and enthusiasm for life

How much sleep is enough sleep? If you would rather go back to bed than get up and start your day, you are not getting enough sleep. If you're feeling tired and would rather take a catnap at 4 p.m. than run another errand, you're not getting enough sleep. When you can't sleep anymore and you're waking up feeling refreshed, that is when you're getting enough sleep. Some people need to take a sleep vacation and give themselves permission to sleep as much as they need for as long as they need. It's not uncommon for someone operating without adequate sleep for many years to sleep twelve to fifteen hours a night for several weeks (once they are provided the time and space to do so) to adequately recharge their batteries.

If you are transitioning away from hyper-palatable foods toward eating real, whole foods, depending on the current state of your health, your body may go through a period of detoxification and withdrawal, in which case you will need more sleep than you've been accustomed to getting. Try to get at least eight hours' sleep, and if possible, if you need more—a lot more—then give yourself permission to get the sleep you need.

Here are a few tips to help you sleep better:

1. **Ditch the alarm**. Try to set up your lifestyle so that you can sleep in and wake up naturally, without an alarm clock. I know this may not be easy, but it is possible.

2. **Get into the groove**. Try adopting a consistent schedule; going to bed and waking up at roughly the same time every day. Sync up your rhythm as much as possible with the natural daylight cycles, going to bed when the sun goes down and waking up with the sun.

3. **Power down**. Many people use electronics very late in the evening, which can prevent melatonin synthesis. Melatonin is a brain chemical that is regulated by light to help you sleep. Light inhibits melatonin production, in effect preventing sleep and causing wakefulness. Try to avoid using electronics at least a couple of hours before bedtime so that melatonin can kick into gear and help you get better quality sleep.

4. **Only for sleeping**. Consider using your bedroom for only sleeping (and lovemaking). Remove all electronics and work-related activities from your bedroom so you can associate your bedroom with bedroom-only activities. Remember, mental associations can be very powerful.

5. **Relax and unwind**. You may want to practice relaxation techniques or meditation in the evening to help you unwind. Providing yourself with ample space and time to recharge your batteries will do you and your body a world of good.

Off the Hook

In addition to eating a real, whole foods diet, meditation, exercise, and adequate sleep can boost the feel-good chemicals in your brain. Taking the time to sit quietly and alone at least once a day, getting a daily dose of physical activity, and affording yourself the luxury of sleep will work wonders to improve your lifestyle. When you step onto this path and start to feel better than you've ever felt before, you may realize is that there is so much more to life, and you can once and for all unhook yourself from the struggle with food.

PART SIX

The Spiritual Hook

"When we look at nutrition from a purely scientific point of view, there is no place for consciousness. And yet, consciousness could be one of the crucial determinants of the metabolism of food itself."

—Deepak Chopra, MD

"Food is unique in that it offers us the tools—both personally and as a community—to transform the most ordinary morsel into the realm of the spiritual and sacred. Eating with mindfulness brings us into the moment, helps us understand what it means to be alive, and connects us to the mystery and source of all living things."

—Donald Altman, *Art of the Inner Meal*

Chapter 11

How Our
Spiritual Isolation Hooks Us

Making the Shift: Eating as a Spiritual Practice

I 'll never forget the day. It was years ago. I sat on my couch watching *The Oprah Winfrey Show*. Oprah's guest was a mother struggling with bulimia. I too was struggling with this eating disorder at that time but did not have the courage to step out in front of millions to reveal it. No, I was hiding away in shame. Her husband and two young boys accompanied her on the show. I couldn't believe how consumed she was with her own disorder. Her sons were expressing their love and "wanted their mom back." They desperately wanted her to love and pay attention to them. She was so blinded by her struggle that she couldn't see that she had a family that cared. She was stuck—hooked on the struggle—and it was consuming her life. In that moment I realized that bulimia was no longer merely a passing problem, but also consumed my life.

When you spend all of your time wrapped up in the struggle with food and your discontent with the size of your thighs or hips, it's as if you're confining yourself to a small dark room with no windows. It's just you, all alone, caught in a mental loop with chronic thoughts of "me and my struggle." Although we don't intend it to be, it can become a very self-absorbed place to live. I thought this way for so many years; it took me a long time to realize that my life's focus was the size of a walnut. My whole life and thought process revolved around feeding my addiction: how to hide it from others, how to pretend to be normal, how to try to keep the weight off, and how to put an end to my suffering.

It wasn't until the most desperate moments of my life, sobbing on the bathroom floor begging the Universe for another chance, that I had realized that this didn't have to be my reality and that I didn't have to choose this to be my life. That moment of insight was like poking my head out from that small dark room to see that there was a vast, open, expansive sky—that there was a whole world going on out there that I wasn't taking part in because I chose to stay hidden away.

The message was loud and clear: when we are caught up in a self-absorbed struggle, we can't wake up to the bigger meaning and purpose of our lives; we stay trapped instead of free. The good news is that your struggle can be an open door to awakening. I also realized that whatever it is we struggle with can, if we so choose, ultimately be what sets us free.

I truly believe that our primary reason for being here is to align with our highest potential and live our joyful life's purpose. I see it everywhere I look; more and more people are awakening to, and aligning with, this heartfelt intention. It is my belief that we are all on a sacred journey, whether we are in tune with that reality or not. Many fundamental perceptual shifts had to take place for me to truly let go of the struggle. I needed to change the way I felt about my body, about food, and about life. From this spiritual perspective —*not* appreciating our bodies or the food we eat, not grasping the miracle of our lives—is the reason we overeat and struggle with food. Because if we saw the magic and beauty inherent in our lives, we wouldn't need to turn to food to manage our distress, because the very purpose of our lives is what nourishes and nurtures our souls.

The Miracle of Our Bodies

I want to offer you a fresh perspective that may shift the way you think about your body. I invite you to suspend all your beliefs, disbeliefs, and recurring thought patterns that no longer serve you—if only for a moment.

"The body is your temple. Keep it pure and clean for the soul to reside in."

—B. K. S. Iyengar

Imagine this: you are here on earth first and foremost having a spiritual experience, and your body is facilitating this experience for you. Lucky you! As one of my favorite authors Wayne Dyer puts it: "Begin to see yourself as a soul with a body rather than a body with a soul." Consider for a moment that we are spiritual beings experiencing this physical plane in physical bodies, and your body is the temple of your consciousness. Your body is the physical manifestation of your soul's desire to experience itself. Your body is your life partner, a companion that you get to share your life with and express your life through—the sacred vessel that is housing your spirit and carrying you on this spiritual journey. Consider yourself the temporary custodian for this temple, responsible for taking care of and maintaining it to its fullest potential as a sign of respect for all life and creation.

Through your body you get to experience what it feels like to hold a baby in your arms, to stand barefoot in the sand, to feel the wind caress your face. You get to taste the wonders of the world through food and smell the fragrances of flowers. You also get to experience a wide range of emotions: falling in love, the sadness of losing a friend, the bittersweet acceptance of letting go of a relationship, the feeling of compassion for someone living on the street.

Your body is a divine miracle, and when you shift your perspective to view it as the miracle that it is, you can start to treat your body with the loving-kindness and respect it deserves. When you build a compassionate relationship with your body that is gentle, open, loving, and kind, you will be better able to listen to what it is communicating to you.

Learning to take loving care of your body is a fundamental part to any spiritual practice and can bring you closer to knowing who you truly are. Paying loving attention to your body is not driven by ego or narcissism but comes from a place of love and gratitude, kindness, and compassion for yourself and this gift that is your body. You'll notice that when you start to take care of your body, it will start taking care of you too; after all, your body is the only place that you have in which to live.

We are literally creating ourselves with the food we eat, the thoughts we think, and the emotions we feel. With this perspective, we become mindful of our thoughts and emotions, and of the food we feed our bodies. Your body works so hard to meet your demands and keep up with your busy agenda; spend time taking care of it and giving it the attention it deserves.

Your body is here to help you through this journey. If you do have a negative body image, I encourage you to shift your perspective to a more loving attitude towards yourself. After all, your body is the most miraculous gift you have been given in this lifetime, and you probably don't want to come to the end of your life wishing that you had realized it sooner.

Pause & Reflect: Making Peace with Your Body

Many of us have been harboring negativity towards our bodies before we can even remember. Making peace with your body may take time, and right now, in this moment, ask yourself if you're willing to embark on this journey to self-love. Connect with your body in some way in this moment. You may want to place your hands on your heart or come back to focusing on your breath. Take the time to slow down and reflect on these questions:

1. Am I ready to accept that my body is a miracle and take responsibility to treat it as such?
2. Am I ready to let go and forgive myself for all the negative ways I've treated my body in the past?
3. Am I ready to know what it feels like to be at peace within my body, mind, and spirit?
4. Am I ready to accept that I no longer have to struggle with food and with my weight, and that I can love and accept myself as I am?

The Miracle of Food

Rather than being a slave who is "hooked" on food, you can become the master of your own destiny. Food can actually serve you and your highest purpose. When you enjoy a harmonious relationship with food, it no longer consumes your energy but in fact frees up your energy; it no longer depletes you but energizes you. Because your relationship with food no longer drains you (as a result of the struggle), you can then turn to more important things in your life, like doing the things you love.

"Food is Spirit. It has come to us through the divine intercourse of heaven and earth. The infinite and eternal cosmic vibrations of light-fire have coalesced and crystallized to form the air, water, earth, plains, all creatures, and us—they are the very heart and soul of us."

—Cecile Tovah Levin, *Cooking for Regeneration*

You have a choice. You can align with food to help fuel your incredible life and support your awakening, or you can engage with food in a way that hinders that process, that gets between you and the life you want to live. Don't you see? It's *your* choice! What reality do you want to live in? When you're caught up in the struggle with food, it's so distracting. That's all you tend to see. When you're free of this struggle—you're *free of the struggle!*

This is the crux of what I'm getting at—how you can align your relationship with food to *support* rather than *hinder* your spiritual journey. I used food as an excuse to hold myself down for many years. I couldn't see beyond my struggle and experience the wonder of life and living because I was so stuck in my struggle with food, my weight, and my distorted body image.

In the search for thinness or the so-called ideal body, many have lost their spiritual connection to food. Realigning your relationship with food allows you to see the divine miracle that it is—pure, life-force potential. We've lost our connection to the miracle of food due to our culture's reductionist mentality that equates food solely to nutrients that can be objectively measured. During processing, the deeper essence of food has been removed along with its life-force. The more we reduce food to singular nutrients, counting calories and calculating grams of fat and carbohydrates, the worse our health gets, and the more people are fixated on food—and the struggle continues.

Analyzing food from an intellectual perspective is not the answer to optimal health, because it's what we *can't* measure in food, the life-giving qualities, that are most important to our health. We don't need more numbers; we need more meaning and significance. We need to look at food as the essence of nourishment.

Life-Force and Pure Love

Ancient and current cultures and traditions all over the world acknowledge the concept of life-force and have adopted it into their cultural perceptions. Hindus recognize this as *prana*. The Chinese call it *chi*. In Hawaiian culture it is referred to as *mana*. Life-force is the energy inherent in all things. It is this energy that enables a tiny seedling to grow into a massive tree and bear fruit. It is what makes our hearts beat—it is the essence of life. Other names for the source of this invisible energy from which all life manifests include God, Creator, Great Spirit, the Divine, or simply Universe. I like to refer to it as Source or Sacred Source, but please insert whatever name most resonates for you.

This Sacred Source is the underlying stillness, the formless place where pure infinite potential resides. All things in existence emanate from Source. It is the birthplace of all thought and creativity, which then translates into physical form. Everything we see in the physical realm was at one point in this formless realm. The house you currently live in was once only a thought in the architect's mind; this book you are holding was once only an idea, a concept in my mind. Source is the vibrant hidden energy that is in everything and that permeates everything. This is the birthplace of all existence. It is pure awareness and pure love energy. We all come from Source and we will all return to Source, the place where nothing begins and nothing ends—it always *is*.

When we align with and tune into this frequency, magical things start to happen; the unfolding of synchronistic events and alignments happen, more creativity flows through us, our intuition strengthens, and we are infused with healing energies.

Food is just one example of the manifestations of this divine life-force in the physical realm, and so are our bodies. In this way, both our bodies and food are life-giving and life-sustaining. This is one of the fundamental ways that we can view nature as being one with us, not separate from us.

In ancient traditions and many indigenous societies, everything ingested in the body was regarded as a sacred communion with this Source energy. Many religions and traditions today still incorporate some level of ceremony around food. Food is revered as a gift from the Earth, as medicine for the totality of our being. There is a conscious awareness around the connectedness of all of life and a deep respect for the land from which the food came. Many cultures have songs and stories about the spirits of individual plants and express deep gratitude to the plants and animals that help them live and thrive. This is spirituality in action.

"Food is a love note from the divine."

—**Gabriel Cousens,** *Spiritual Nutrition*

Embodying What We Eat

In the moment that we eat, a transformation takes place—we embody the energies of our food. When we eat, we are literally assimilating and merging the outer world with our inner world. We become one with and resonate with the frequencies of the earth; a remarkable transferring of energy from the earth into our being. Eating life-force gives us life-force; the more "alive" the food is, the higher the life-force inherent in it. It is this life-force that wakes up our consciousness. The information inherent in this life-force floods every single cell of our body, and the basis of this information is life-giving, life-supporting, and life-enhancing. The energy of the earth can penetrate every single cell of your body and whisper messages of growth and vitality. Source carries a vibration of pure love, and food is a manifestation from this Divine realm. When we choose to eat foods straight from Source, directly from Mother Earth, this enables us to align with the vibrations of this pure-love frequency.

That's why I choose to eat as close to nature as possible, and I mean that both physically and metaphorically. When we eat real, whole food, we embody this pure energy source. Each bite we take of real food is an opportunity that brings us closer to and aligns us with our original nature. When we eat processed foods, we create an energy deficit by trying to process something foreign to our bodies. Even beyond that, we embody the energy that makes up the industry that produced that food, an industry that revolves around greed, fear, competition, and addiction. When we don't eat in a way that nurtures our bodies with life-giving nutrients, we tend to feel lethargic, sluggish, anxious, and moody. Toxicity literally blocks the flow of energy coming through our bodies and weakens our bodies, minds, and spirits.

Once you start to eat real, whole foods, your relationship with food will naturally shift, and you will notice what a pleasure food can be; food will become a source of joy, not pain. Then you can return to your roots of connectedness, of gratitude for the earth, not only benefiting yourself but others as well. When you eat and connect to the gifts of nourishment you receive, you can then nourish others in return—through helping others or serving your highest purpose. Either way, you are allowing the creative life-force to flow through you.

The Power of Connection

The way we eat is intricately connected to our spiritual life. When we take the time to connect with food, we see that everything is deeply interconnected.

"The food we eat can reveal the interconnectedness of the universe, the earth, all living beings, and ourselves."

—Thich Nhat Hanh

When you truly understand, not from a conceptual level but from a feeling level, that the same invisible life-force that runs through you runs through everything else—every ant, every flower, every bird, every blade of grass—and you realize how connected we all are, then you can start to live your life from this

Chapter 12

Unhooked: Deepening Your Spiritual Connection

Many of the practices we've discussed in this book can strengthen the connection to our spiritual selves. The simple act of paying attention to what we eat can open us up to be in awe of the many mysteries of life. Meditation, the practice of loving-kindness, mindful eating, moving your body through joyful movement, and developing self-compassion all provide a solid foundation for anyone ready to leave the struggle with food behind and walk the path of awakening to their highest self. In this final chapter, I would like to offer one more tool for you to take with you on your journey: the practice of cultivating gratitude and appreciation. It's easy to forget how special the miracle of life is in our busy, consumerist culture, where we tend to focus on what we don't have and what we want to acquire. Incorporating the simple, humble practice of gratitude and making it the foundation upon which you build everything else can transform your life.

When you move toward a "feeling space" of true, heartfelt gratitude, you change the frequency you are tuning into, connecting to the healing, pure-love frequency of our Sacred Source and to your inherent wisdom. When you tune into this channel, your body, mind, and spirit are in harmony. This is the space where we experience joy, peace, and freedom from struggle.

The Healing Power of Gratitude

Science now supports what the mystics have known for millennia: our minds and bodies are not separate but intricately interconnected. Feeling positive emotions is good for our bodies on a physical level, and the contrary holds true as well. Perpetuating negative emotions doesn't do any*body* good.

"When you realize there is nothing lacking, the whole world belongs to you."

—Lao Tzu

Gratitude is the quality of being thankful and appreciative. Expressing gratitude is another instant way to shift towards a more positive emotional state and naturally boost the feel good chemicals in the brain. Ever noticed that feelings of gratitude and appreciation can instantly make you feel better? How we choose to focus our attention and the mental attitude we choose to show up with day in and day out have huge implications for our health. When we focus on heart-centered feelings like gratitude, actual physical changes take place in our bodies. According to physician and author Christiane Northrup, practicing gratitude can decrease stress hormones, relax coronary arteries, allow us to breathe deeper, and increase blood supply to the heart, raising the level of oxygen supply to the tissues.[136]

Scientists at the Institute of HeartMath, an organization that researches the effects of "core heart feelings" like gratitude on our bodies, have found that positive and negative emotions have very different effects on the body, particularly the autonomic nervous system (ANS).[137] As discussed in chapter 8, the ANS is the part of the peripheral nervous system that regulates, among other things, involuntary body functions such as digestion, heartbeat, breathing, and secretion of hormones. The ANS is divided into the sympathetic nervous system (fight or flight) and the parasympathetic nervous system (rest and relax).

Emotional states like anger, depression, stress, and jealousy can lead to a change in the body's heart rhythm and activate the sympathetic nervous system, adversely affecting the rest of the body. Disharmony in the ANS leads to inefficiency and increased stress on the heart and other organs and reduces the optimal functioning capacity of the body overall.

On the other hand, positive emotions create physiological benefits in the body. Positive emotions such as gratitude and appreciation, compassion, love, and kindness create increased harmony and coherence in heart rhythms, causing more efficiency and less stress to the body's systems and overall functioning. This affects everything—from our mental capacities to our digestive function.[138]

Exercise #1: Practice On-the-Spot Gratitude

For a simple and effective way to shift to your heart center and reap the many physical, mental, and emotional benefits of tuning into and fostering positive emotions, follow these three simple steps:

1. Shift your attention from your mind to your heart by focusing on your heart center. Use your hand to help you focus your attention by placing one or both of your hands over your heart.
2. Breathe into your heart center. Focus on your heart while you breathe. Imagine that your breath is literally being inhaled and exhaled directly through your chest into your heart.
3. Name something you are grateful for: a person, place, opportunity, body part, pet, whole food, children, etc. Feel the love, gratitude, and appreciation that you have for this in your life. Breathe into it and rest here for as long as you like. You've just shifted your physiological response to one that is more efficient and resonant with the vibration of gratitude.

Keep a Gratitude Journal

Keeping a gratitude journal was my first gratitude practice. I was eighteen and very depressed, and I was told I should go on antidepressants. I knew this wasn't a solution for me, and luckily, soon afterward, I heard someone talking about the benefits of gratitude when feeling depressed. I tried it, and it worked wonders for me, helping me through a very difficult time in my life—minus all the side effects that antidepressants may have caused.[*]

---

[*] Please consult your health care practitioner if you are considering going off any medication.

Gratitude journaling is a great technique for managing stress, coping with difficult situations, and spending some quiet time alone. It doesn't have to be forced or complicated; just start with anything for which you genuinely feel grateful for. I simply wrote down three things I was grateful for, every morning and night. At first it was hard to feel appreciation because I was so down on myself. But over time, as the list grew, it got easier to find things I was truly grateful for: a cozy bed to sleep in, the love and support of my family, a special conversation, or spending time with my cuddly cat. This became a priceless resource for me. I could pick up my gratitude journal and instantly be reminded of all that I have to be grateful for and how special life is.

Gratitude for Your Body

It was a special day. I was in elementary school, and we were invited to listen to an inspirational guest speaker; this meant we were skipping class. I don't remember his name, but I do remember he didn't have arms, and I especially remember that he drove himself to our school. I looked down at my hands and experienced one of my earliest memories of gratitude toward my body. It had never occurred to me before; some people *didn't* have hands, and I just so happened to be lucky enough to have them.

Growing up, the moments I felt genuine gratitude for my body were few and far between. More often than not I was consumed with self-critical thoughts toward my body for not being thinner, firmer, smoother, stronger, darker, and prettier. At times, I feel as if I'm still healing from all those years of self-criticism. One of the ways I've made amends with my body and learned to accept this gift I've been given is through gratitude practices, specifically towards my body.

Exercise #2: Body Gratitude Practice: Thank Your Feet

There are a number of ways that you can practice connecting to a heartfelt appreciation for your body. This "Thank Your Feet" practice allows you to start with a feeling toward your body that you can easily and genuinely connect to and then naturally expand out to other parts of your body that you might find more difficult to love, embrace, and fully accept.

1. Get comfortable either sitting or lying down. If you lie down, prop your head up on a pillow so you can see your bare feet and toes.

2. Look at your feet. Take the time to really look at them as if seeing them for the first time. Examine all the little crevices and curves and spaces between your toes.

3. Think about what your life would be like if you didn't have your feet. Think about the convenience, opportunity, and experiences these feet have provided you. Your feet have carried you every single step of this incredible journey. Isn't this an amazing thought to contemplate?

4. Thank your feet for the gift that they are. You can either simply rest with this feeling or, if you're ready to break down old negative thought patterns about your body, keep going.

5. Move your attention to a part of your body that you've been less than grateful for. It could be your thighs, your behind, your nose, your hair, or your arms—whatever part of your body that you've struggled with accepting and loving. Take a moment to connect to this part of your body. Imagine what it would be like not to have your nose or any hair at all, or to not have thighs. Send this part of your body love. Imagine the cells in this part of your body radiating light. With an attitude of self-compassion, thank this body part for supporting your life experience. Notice what comes up for you when you practice this. Is it easier or perhaps more difficult than you thought?

Gratitude for Food

Gratitude was an essential practice that helped propel a drastic shift in my relationship with food. Because we eat every day, and food is so available everywhere we look, it's easy to forget what a special gift each bite of real, whole food is. This practice has ushered me into a new reality where I have deep reverence for the divine essence of the foods I eat.

I'm constantly in awe of the way the earth nourishes plants, and the way these plants, in turn, nourish my being to grow and develop. When you are grateful for the food in front of you, it's hard not to realize that this food is what's giving you life, which in turn enhances our reverence towards foods. This is how our relationship with food can infuse our lives with deeper purpose and meaning.

There are many ways we can express our gratitude for food, and one of my favorites is through honoring meals with a mealtime blessing.

"Because food is what it is, it is of utmost importance that we receive it with deep gratitude, because we consume life. Whether it's cabbage or cows, it's life that we consume . . . . How can we not be grateful for the life that sustains us?"

—**John Daido Loori**, Zen master

Blessing Your Food

Giving thanks by blessing your food before you eat is another way to help you connect to the sacredness in your everyday life. When you shift your perception to remember the true miracle that food is, it's easy to give thanks before you eat. Expressing gratitude for your food goes hand in hand with the mindfulness practices outlined in chapter 8 on mindful eating. To eat with gratitude is to eat with awareness. It's more difficult to be grateful when eating while distracted in front of the television or eating on the run. Blessing your food before you eat is another mindful eating technique that you can use to slow things down and allow time to center yourself before you begin to eat. This pause offers time for contemplation and an opportunity to connect with gratitude and the deeper meaning of your food.

Consider offering a blessing both at the beginning and the end of your meal. When you say a blessing before you eat, it sets a special tone for the meal. When you end with a blessing, it punctuates the meal with appreciation, as it allows you to gratefully acknowledge that you just ate. It can be as simple as "Thank you for this meal," or you can choose to connect to our common humanity and offer a blessing like, "May all beings be fed and nourished with whole foods."

Mealtime blessings can be done in many different ways. Find what works for you. You can say a blessing anytime, anywhere, with any food, with or without people present. You can say a blessing out loud or in silence. When you bless your food while eating with others, it creates a sense of community, starting together and ending together, and creates a shared experience of gratitude. When eating in a group, one person may volunteer to say a blessing, or perhaps everyone can take a turn to say one thing they are grateful for as you go around the circle. As a group, you may choose to eat in silence or perhaps start the meal in silence, allowing quiet space to fully appreciate the conscious act of eating.

There are many different aspects of food that you can be grateful for. You may choose to focus on a specific theme or just let it flow freely. You can also bless your food with a song or a chant, as my husband and I like to do. You can give thanks for the elements that supported the growth and creation of the food, the colors of the food and all the nutrients in the food, or all the people who participated in bringing this meal to the table.

Blessing your food is a mindful eating practice that can help you end your struggle with food, because it allows you to broaden your perspective and become aware of the connectedness that everything and everyone shares. When you don't feel connected, you are more prone to disrespect the earth, yourself, and your body. Gratitude allows you to honor the food you eat and thus honor yourself, changing the way you relate to food and the relationship you have with food. This is how food can become a part of your spiritual practice.

Here is an example of a mealtime blessing I use:

"I bless this food and put it in my body with positive intention. I have appreciation and gratitude for the hands that helped bring this food before me. This food is infused with energy from the sun and is filled with nutrients from the earth and water, connected to all living beings. I use the energy from this food to create a life filled with joy for myself and all others."

Vietnamese Buddhist monk and teacher Thich Nhat Hanh offers this approach to blessing food, incorporating gratitude throughout the whole process of eating.[139]

1. **Serving food:** In this food I see clearly the presence of the entire universe supporting my existence.
2. **Looking at the filled plate:** All living beings are struggling for life. May they all have enough food to eat today.
3. **Just before eating:** The plate is filled with food. I am aware that each morsel is the fruit of much hard work by those who produced it.
4. **Beginning to eat:** With the first taste, I promise to practice loving-kindness. With the second, I promise to relieve the suffering of others. With the third, I promise to see others' joy as my own.

With the fourth, I promise to learn the way of non-attachment and equanimity.

5. **Finishing the meal:** The plate is empty. My hunger is satisfied. I vow to live for the benefit of all beings.

These mealtime rituals help us to remember that we are connected to our food. It is easier to feel connected when acting connected. Be aware of what is on your plates, where it comes from, and ask how your food choices are affecting those around you and our planet. Try to walk mindfully and respectfully on this earth with gratitude for all of these divine gifts that we've been given. This is what it means to live with a heart filled with gratitude.

Pause & Reflect: Discovering Your Life's Purpose

By this time, you can see that your struggle with food is about so much more than just food and how much you weigh. This is about your life, and the way that you chose to live it. Take as long as you like to pause and reflect on these final questions:

1. Am I ready to live the life I've always dreamed of? If not, what's stopping me?
2. Am I ready to accept responsibility for the vision of my life?
3. Am I ready to move on from the old ways of being and let go of outdated belief systems?
4. Am I ready to accept and trust that I deserve happiness, and that I am worthy of all the goodness in my life?
5. Am I ready to align with what I really want to experience and manifest in this lifetime?

Unhooked: What Are You Really Hungry For?

When we stand back and look at the bigger picture, we can see that there are many interconnected reasons we continuously turn to food for more than sustenance. We know that the primary reason we eat is because we're hungry, yet our relationship with food extends far beyond that. It incorporates aspects of our physiology, emotions, behaviors, and thought patterns, all rooted in a culture that supports and fosters an unhealthy, disordered relationship with food.

Our environment is geared towards overconsumption, and the foods that are most abundant and readily accessible are highly addictive and evoke powerful emotional responses within us. At times, life can be difficult; no one is immune to the challenges and struggles of life. Food offers us pleasure, a temporary moment of relief, a time-out from the stress and chaos. It gets more complicated when we then turn to foods that produce a hyper-pleasurable response in us, a quick and legal fix to help get us through the day. We then become habituated, and these behavioral patterns become reinforced and strengthened. Many people become hooked on this cycle, falling into patterns of binging and restricting, struggling to find balance and peace within their cravings.

There's more to life than being caught in the continuous, reinforcing feedback loop of our struggle with food. Our spiritual selves yearn for something far greater than the instant and fleeting pleasure that comes from satisfying a craving. Many people have been caught in this struggle with food because they have been using food as a means of distraction and as a way to fill a void within themselves, a void that can only be nourished with love, with *purpose.*

Breaking free from the struggle starts with returning to real, whole foods and seeing the true miracle that these foods are. Discovering joyful movement like walking, spending time in nature, connecting with your food source, and fostering gratitude and appreciation for the miracle of life—these are ways that you can nourish and nurture your spirit. Spending quiet time alone every day in meditation or contemplation will also be invaluable to you on this journey; so will fostering strong, healthy social connections. Do what makes you feel good: dance or listen to music, get a daily dose of sun, treat yourself to a nice long bath or a massage. You can learn to manage your stress by remembering not to take yourself so seriously and find the humor and irony in life. Watch the miracle of life unfold before your eyes. You only have one life to live: do you want to spend your whole life caught in an endless struggle that only brings you more suffering? Try to adopt an attitude of self-compassion and loving-kindness; be gentle on yourself, and forgive yourself. And most importantly, ask yourself:

"What am I really hungry for?"

What brings you a true, lasting sense of contentment, of satisfaction, peace, and joy? Is it really food? Or is it spending time with your children, or helping someone else in need? Is it taking time for yourself, or perhaps doing work that you're passionate about and brings meaning into your life? You know what you love: *go there*, follow that feeling . . . wherever that leads you.

Appendix A

Yale Food Addiction Scale

Am I Struggling with an Addiction to Food?

Take a moment to reflect on the following questions from the Yale Food Addiction Scale developed by Ashley Gearhardt of Yale University. This questionnaire is based on the seven criteria of substance dependence and is scientifically validated. This is a quick and easy, abbreviated version of the Yale Food Addiction Scale (used with permission).

The Yale Food Addiction Scale (Abbreviated)

The following questions ask about your eating habits in the past year. People sometimes have difficulty controlling their intake of certain foods such as sweets, starches, salty snacks, fatty foods, sugary drinks, and others.

Please answer the following seven questions using this scale:

0: Never
1: Once per month
2: 2–4 times per month
3: 2–3 times per week
4: 4+ times per week

	Question:	Answer
1.	I find myself consuming certain foods even though I am no longer hungry.	
2.	I worry about cutting down on certain foods.	
3.	I feel sluggish or fatigued from overeating.	
4.	I have spent time dealing with negative feelings from overeating certain foods, instead of spending time in important activities such as time with family, friends, work, or recreation.	
5.	I have had physical withdrawal symptoms such as agitation and anxiety when I cut down on certain foods. (Do not include caffeinated drinks: coffee, tea, cola, energy drinks, etc.)	
6.	My behavior with respect to food and eating causes me significant distress.	
7.	Issues related to food and eating decrease my ability to function effectively (daily routine, job/school, social or family activities, health difficulties).	
8.	In the past 12 months... I kept consuming the same types or amounts of food despite significant emotional and/or physical problems related to my eating.	YES ☐ or NO ☐
9.	In the past 12 months... Eating the same amount of food does not reduce negative emotions or increase pleasurable feelings the way it used to.	YES ☐ or NO ☐

Scoring

If your answers matched at least three of the following scores, you may meet the criteria for food addiction:

Question 1: 4
Question 2: 4
Question 3: 3 or 4
Question 4: 3 or 4
Question 5: 3 or 4
Question 6: 3 or 4
Question 7: 3 or 4
AND answered "Yes" to either question 8 or 9, or both.
Question 8: Yes
Question 9: Yes

Understanding Fruit Sugars: Glycemic Index Versus Glycemic Load

Many health professionals advise people not to eat fruit because it's too high in sugar and will cause blood sugar disorders. Let's look at one of the key measurements of carbohydrates in relation to blood sugar to gain a better understanding.

The *glycemic index* (GI) is a numerical scale used to indicate how fast a carbohydrate-containing food can raise blood sugar levels. The consumption of high-GI foods results in more rapid increases in blood glucose levels than the consumption of low-GI foods. Both too much and not enough sugar in the blood is problematic; that's why the body has built-in mechanisms to keep blood sugar levels within a specific range. The physical manifestations of high and low blood sugar levels are found in hyperglycemia and hypoglycemia, respectively. A GI score for a food of 70 or more is considered high (it will raise blood glucose levels very fast), a GI of 56 to 69 is medium, and a GI of 55 or less is low.

But the GI is only part of the story. The GI may tell us how quickly a food can increase blood sugar, but it doesn't tell us by how much, which is determined by the *quantity* of carbohydrates in a serving of that particular food. Glycemic index measures quality, so we need another tool to measure quantity. This is where the glycemic load comes into play.

The *glycemic load* (GL) has more recently been adopted into mainstream use. Used in conjunction with the GI, the GL paints a more complete and accurate picture of the role that carbohydrates (sugars) play in our bloodstream and the extent to which they influence blood sugar levels. To gain the best understanding, we need to look at both quality (GI) and quantity (GL). The GL is calculated by multiplying a food's glycemic index value by the amount of available carbohydrates per serving, which means subtracting grams of fiber from grams of carbohydrates.

Watermelon is a great example. Watermelon often comes under attack for being a high-sugar food, and despite the discrepancies found in various GI rating scales, watermelon consistently ranks as "high" on the glycemic index (although most fruits consistently rank low to medium on the GI).

But how much sugar is actually in watermelon? How much would we have to eat to get an abnormally large spike in blood sugar? Because watermelon is so high in water content and fiber, there's actually not a lot of sugar in one single serving, so despite having a high GI score it comes in relatively low in the GL score (GI = 72; GL = 4). As we discussed in chapter 4, fruits have a built in mechanism (fiber and water) to prevent overconsumption and help normalize the rate of glucose absorption.

The vast majority of fruits fall into either the low or medium category on both the GI and GL scale, with few exceptions. As soon as we start refining the carbohydrates and concentrating them into condensed forms of sugar (this includes all refined, processed foods), this changes how they affect blood sugar levels. This also applies to dried fruits and fruit juices. Many people still consider dried fruit to be a whole food, but how can it be whole when we've removed all the water content? With fruit juices, the fiber has been removed. Although dried fruits and juices may be a healthier alternative to eating refined sugars, they are still not a whole food and are not as optimal as eating whole fruits with the water and fiber content intact. Whenever possible, reach for whole, organic fruits and vegetables.

Appendix C

Basic Sitting Practice: Mindfulness-Awareness Meditation

This meditation practice is also called mindfulness-awareness practice. I encourage you to seek out the many resources available to help guide you on your journey, including the audio course *How to Meditate with Pema Chödrön: A Practical Guide to Making Friends with Your Mind* produced by Sounds True.

Remember to surround your practice with the qualities of loving-kindness and gentleness, curiosity, humor, patience, and compassion. These qualities allow you to lighten up and take a softer approach, and connect to the relaxed dimension of your being as you learn to let go of rigidity and fixed ways of being and thinking. Approaching your feelings and emotions with these qualities creates a safe space for you to connect with the present moment.

1. Find a comfortable place to sit, with minimal distractions.

2. If you are using a cushion, make sure you are level, not leaning in any one direction. If this is uncomfortable, you may want to allow your pelvis to tilt slightly forward, helping your knees to relax to the floor. If you can't sit comfortably on the floor or on a cushion, sit in a chair that allows you to sit with a straight back, both feet comfortably on the floor.

3. If sitting on the floor, fold your legs comfortably in front of you. Avoid crossing your ankles to avoid pressure on your joints. Instead place one ankle in front of the other on the floor.

4. Find the center on your sitting bones. You can do this by gently rocking side-to-side and front-to-back and then come back to center.

5. Sit with your torso upright but relaxed. This helps to create space for your internal organs. The main focus here is that the front of your body is open and not slumped or crouched. You can do this by rolling your shoulders up, back, and down. This allows your heart space to open up.

6. Elongate your spine by pushing the crown of your head towards the ceiling. Imagine that there is a string coming out from the top of your head, and it is pulling you upwards. Be mindful to not arch your back, as this will create stress on the body. You can check your lower back by placing your hand on your lower back and adjusting accordingly, making sure it's in line with your tailbone.

7. Adjust your neck so that the back of your neck is long and relaxed, with your chin slightly tucked in.

8. Rest your hands comfortably, palms facing downwards on your thighs.

9. Your eyes are slightly open with a soft gaze. Your eye gaze is slightly downward, four to six feet in front of you.

10. Mouth is relaxed, jaw is slightly open, and you can rest the tip of the tongue on the front roof of the mouth. Relax your forehead, your facial muscles, your eyes, and your neck.

Once you get comfortable in your posture, simply begin to notice. Although it is simple, it can also be challenging. Paying attention can be difficult, because we are used to constant distraction. There are two techniques surrounding your breath and thoughts that can help you learn how to pay attention and remind you to keep coming back to your pure, open awareness.

Breath: Your Primary Focus

Allow yourself to notice your breath, and simply breathe naturally and easily. Breath goes out and breath comes in, not being forced in any one direction. The breath is the basis of this practice, a technique to bring you back to the present moment. It's the anchor point that allows you to continuously return to a point of focus. Think of it as home base. Having this anchor point helps you to notice how often you mentally "leave," and you will slowly begin to gain greater appreciation for the description "learning to stay present." Through this practice, you learn to return to home base over and over again. Inevitably you will start to realize how many times you continuously turn away from the present moment throughout your day. With every breath we repeatedly learn to let go and embrace our ever-changing reality. We learn how to deeply relax with who we are.

Thoughts: Like Clouds in the Sky

The first thing people tend to notice once they start practicing this mindfulness-awareness technique is how busy their minds are. As you learn to meditate, you will also notice that your thoughts won't stop coming and going, although some people experience busier minds than others. However busy your mind is on any given day, it will increasingly become within your control to choose if you get hooked and swept away by your thoughts, or simply witness them as an observer, as if watching a movie on a screen. As much as you can, simply acknowledge the thoughts in a relaxed, gentle, kind, and non-judgmental way. Every time you notice a thought, say to yourself, "thinking," and then relax your focus and return your attention to your breath.

One way that you can make friends with your thoughts is to think of them as clouds in the vast openness of the sky. The clouds come and go, again and again, and you simply watch them pass. When you see a cloud, imagine that you can reach up and gently touch it as you say "thinking" to yourself, and then return to the breath. "Touch" the cloud with loving-kindness and gentleness as you see it dissolve and evaporate. If your thoughts are like clouds, then your mind is like the vast openness of the sky. With meditation you can learn how to connect with this vast openness, which is the true nature of your mental landscape.

About the Author

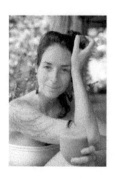

Laura Dawn is a Holistic Health Consultant, Raw Food Chef and is also the author of "Mindful Eating for Dummies". After discovering the secrets to healing her disordered eating, Laura Dawn has inspired others to drop their struggle with food and weight. A dynamic keynote speaker, her passion is to inspire people to choose a sustainable path of health and happiness. She is the founder of Happy & Raw (www.happyandraw. com) and runs health retreats in Hawaii, where she resides on her organic farm.

Endnotes

1   Anne Katherine, *Anatomy of a Food Addiction: The Brain Chemistry of Overeating* (Gurze Books, 1991).

2   David Kessler, Authors@Google, May 28, 2009, http://www.youtube.com/watch?v=A7M_mqXzpr8

3   Fritjof Capra, *The Web of Life: A New Scientific Understanding of Living Systems* (Anchor Books, 1996), 19.

4   Fritjof Capra, *The Web of Life*, 29.

5   See http://www.kraftbrands.com/sites/KraftNutrition/PDF/knu-Article-For-Professionals-08-Spring.pdf.

6   Michael Moss, *Salt Sugar Fat: How the Food Giants Hooked Us* (Random House, 2013), 126.

7   Michael Moss, *Salt Sugar Fat: How the Food Giants Hooked Us*, 126.

8   L. Vartanian, C. Herman, and B. Wansink, "Are We Aware of the External Factors That Influence Food Intake?" *Health Psychology* 27, no. 5 (2008): 533–538.

9   Brian Wansink, "Environmental Factors That Increase the Food Intake and Consumption Volume of Unknowing Consumers," 2004, http://foodpsychology.cornell.edu/pdf/permission/2004/EnvironCues-ARN_2004.pdf.

10   C. P. Herman, D. A. Roth, and J. Polivy, "Effects of the Presence of Others on Eating: A Normative Interpretation," *Psychological Bulletin* 129 (2003): 873–886.

11   C. P. Herman, S. Koenig-Nobert, J. B. Peterson, and J. Polivy, "Matching Effects on Eating: Do Individual Differences Make a Difference?" *Appetite* 45 (2005): 108–109.

12   J. M. de Castro and E. M. Brewer, "The Amount Eaten in Meals by Humans Is a Power Function of the Number of People Present," *Physiology & Behavior* 51 (1992): 121–125.

13   Brian Wansink, James E. Painter, and Yeon-Kyung Lee, "The Office Candy Dish: Proximity's Influence on Estimated and Actual Consumption," *International Journal of Obesity* 30.5 (2006): 871–875.

14   B. Wansink, J. E. Painter, and J. North, "Bottomless Bowls: Why Visual Cues of Portion Size May Influence Intake," *Obesity Research* 13 (2005): 93–100.

15   H. Raynor and L. Epstein, "Dietary Variety, Energy Regulation, and Obesity," *Psychological Bulletin* 127 (2001): 325–341.

16   Barbara J. Rolls, Edward A. Rowe, Edmund T. Rolls, Breda Kingston, Angela Megson, and Rachel Gunary, "Variety in a Meal Enhances Food Intake in Man," *Physiology and Behavior* 26 (1981): 215–21.

17   See http://www.foodpsychology.cornell.edu/research/summary-popcorn. html.

18   L. Smolak and M. P. Levine, eds. *The Developmental Psychopathology of Eating Disorders: Implications for Research, Prevention, and Treatment* (Lawrence Erlbaum Associates, Inc., 1996).

19   H. W. Hoek, "The Distribution of Eating Disorders," in K. D. Brownell and C.G. Fairburn, eds., *Eating Disorders and Obesity: A Comprehensive Handbook* (Guilford, 1995), 207–211.

20   L. Smolak, National Eating Disorders Association/Next Door Neighbors Puppet Guide Book, 1996.

21   See http://ns.umich.edu/new/releases/6892.

22   Deakin University (Melbourne, Australia), "Healthy Parks, Healthy People: The Health Benefits of Contact with Nature in a Park," March 2008, http:// parkweb.vic.gov.au/__data/assets/pdf_file/0018/313821/HPHP-deakin- literature-review.pdf.

23   Clinton Ober, Stephen T. Sinatra, and Martin Zucker, *Earthing: The Most Important Health Discovery Ever?* (Basic Health Publications Inc., 2010).

24   Clinton Ober, Stephen T. Sinatra, and Martin Zucker, *Earthing: The Most Important Health Discovery Ever?*

25   Nicholas A. Christakis and James H. Fowler, "The Spread of Obesity in a Large Social Network Over 32 Years," *New England Journal of Medicine* 357 (2007): 370–379.

26   Nicholas A. Christakis and James H. Fowler, "Dynamic Spread of Happiness in a Large Social Network: Longitudinal Analysis over 20 Years in the Framingham Heart Study," *British Medical Journal* 337 (2008): 2338.

27   Fiona M. Alpass and S. Neville, "Loneliness, Health, and Depression in Older Males," *Aging & Mental Health* 7, no. 3 (2003): 212–216.

28   Avshalom Caspi, HonaLee Harrington, Terrie E. Moffitt, Barry J. Milne, and Richie Poulton, "Socially Isolated Children 20 Years Later: Risk of Cardiovascular Disease," *Archives of Pediatrics & Adolescent Medicine* 160, no. 8 (2006): 805.

29   Michael Moss, *Salt Sugar Fat*, 10.

30   Michael Lutter and Eric J. Nestler, "Homeostatic and Hedonic Signals Interact in the Regulation of Food Intake," *The Journal of Nutrition* 139.3 (2009): 629–632.

31   Alice V. Ely, Samantha Winter, and Michael R. Lowe, "The Generation and Inhibition of Hedonically Driven Food Intake: Behavioral and Neurophysiological Determinants in Healthy Weight Individuals," *Physiology & Behavior* (2013).

32   Kenneth Blum, et al, "Reward Circuitry Dopaminergic Activation Regulates Food and Drug Craving Behavior," *Current Pharmaceutical Design* 17.12 (2011): 1158–1167.

33   Magalie Lenoir, Fuschia Serre, Lauriane Cantin, and Serge H. Ahmed, "Intense Sweetness Surpasses Cocaine Reward," PLOS ONE 2, no. 8 (2007): e698.

34   Gene-Jack Wang, et al. "Imaging of Brain Dopamine Pathways: Implications for Understanding Obesity," *Journal of Addiction Medicine* 3.1 (2009): 8.

35   See http://www.foodaddiction.com/Publications/SciencePage5.html

36   Anne Katherine, *Anatomy of a Food Addiction*, 25.

37   Anne Katherine, *Anatomy of a Food Addiction*, 40.

38   David A. Kessler, *The End of Overeating: Taking Control of the Insatiable American Appetite* (Rodale Books, 2009), 10.

39   David A. Kessler, *The End of Overeating.*

40   Nora D. Volkow, et al. "Inverse Association between BMI and Prefrontal Metabolic Activity in Healthy Adults," *Obesity* 17.1 (2008): 60–65.

41   Alice V. Ely, Samantha Winter, and Michael R. Lowe, "The Generation and Inhibition of Hedonically Driven Food Intake: Behavioral and Neurophysiological Determinants in Healthy Weight Individuals," *Physiology & Behavior* (2013).

42   Douglas Graham, *The 80/10/10 Diet: Balancing Your Health, Your Weight, and Your Life One Luscious Bite at a Time* (FoodnSport Press, 2006), 83.

43   Yunsheng Ma, Barbara Olendzki, David Chiriboga, James R. Hebert, Youfu Li, Wenjun Li, MaryJane Campbell, Katherine Gendreau, and Ira S. Ockene, "Association between Dietary Carbohydrates and Body Weight," *American Journal of Epidemiology* 161, no. 4 (2005): 359–367.

44   Lee S. Gross, Li Li, Earl S. Ford, and Simin Liu, "Increased Consumption of Refined Carbohydrates and the Epidemic of Type 2 Diabetes in the United States: An Ecologic Assessment," *American Journal of Clinical Nutrition* 79, no. 5 (2004): 774–779.

45   S. Liu, W. C. Willett, M. J. Stampfer, et al. "A Prospective Study of Dietary Glycemic Load, Carbohydrate Intake, and Risk of Coronary Heart Disease in US Women. *American Journal of Clinical Nutrition* 71, no. 6 (2000): 1455–61.

46   J. R. Thornton, P. M. Emmett, and K. W. Heaton, "Diet and Crohn's Disease: Characteristics of the Pre-Illness Diet," *British Medical Journal* 2, no. 6193 (1979): 762.

47   L. S. A. Augustin, L. Dal Maso, C. La Vecchia, M. Parpinel, E. Negri, S. Vaccarella, C. W. C. Kendall, D. J. A. Jenkins, and S. Franceschi, "Dietary Glycemic Index and Glycemic Load, and Breast Cancer Risk: A Case-Control Study," *Annals of Oncology* 12, no. 11 (2001): 1533–1538.

48   S. Franceschi, L. Dal Masco, L. Augustin, E. Negri, M. Parpinel, P. Boyle, D. J. A. Jenkins, and C. La Vecchia. "Dietary Glycemic Load and Colorectal Cancer Risk," *Annals of Oncology* 12, no. 2 (2001): 173–178.

49   Larry Christensen, "Effects of Eating Behavior on Mood: A Review of the Literature," *International Journal of Eating Disorders* 14, no. 2 (1993): 171–183.

50   Joshua P. Thaler, Chun-Xia Yi, Ellen A. Schur, Stephan J. Guyenet, Bang H.
      Hwang, Marcelo O. Dietrich, Xiaolin Zhao, et al. "Obesity Is Associated
      with Hypothalamic Injury in Rodents and Humans," *The Journal of Clinical
      Investigation* 122, no. 1 (2012): 153.

51   Douglas Graham, *The 80/10/10 Diet*, 32.

52   Elson Haas with Buck Levin, *Staying Healthy With Nutrition: The Complete
      Guide to Diet and Nutritional Medicine*, (Celestial Arts, 2006), 173.

53   See http://www.cdc.gov/salt/pdfs/Salt_Stats_Media.pdf.

54   David B. Young, H. U. A. B. A. O. Lin, and Richard D. McCabe,
      "Potassium's Cardiovascular Protective Mechanisms," *American Journal of
      Physiology—Regulatory, Integrative, and Comparative Physiology* 268.4 (1995):
      R825–R837.

55   Panel on Dietary Reference Intakes for Electrolytes and Water, Standing
      Committee on the Scientific Evaluation of Dietary Reference Intakes;
      Dietary Reference Intakes for Water, Potassium, Sodium, Chloride, and Sulfate
      (The National Academies Press, 2005).

56   W. Koszewski, "How Much Sodium Are You Eating?" University of
      Nebraska-Lincoln Extension, http://www.ianrpubs.unl.edu/epublic/pages/
      publicationD.jsp?publicationId=1223.

57   Report of the Dietary Guidelines Advisory Committee on the Dietary
      Guidelines for Americans, United States Department of Agriculture, Center
      for Nutrition Policy and Promotion, 2010.

58   Strategies to Reduce Sodium Intake in the United States, Institute of
      Medicine, April 2010, http://www.iom.edu/~/media/Files/Report%20
      Files/2010/Strategies-to-Reduce-Sodium-Intake-in-the-United States/
      Strategies%20to%20Reduce%20Sodium%20Intake%202010%20%20
      Report%20Brief.ashx.

59   Elson Haas with Buck Levin, *Staying Healthy With Nutrition*, 172.

60   Matthew T. Gailliot and Roy F. Baumeister, "The Physiology of Willpower:
      Linking Blood Glucose to Self-Control," *Personality and Social Psychology
      Review* 11, no. 4 (2007): 303–327.

61   I credit the phrase "whole, fresh, ripe, raw, organic plants" to Dr. Douglas
      Graham.

62   H. Boeing, A. Bechthold, A. Bub, S. Ellinger, D. Haller, A. Kroke, E.
      Leschik-Bonnet, M. J. Müller, H. Oberritter, M. Schulze, P. Stehle, and B.

Watzl, "Critical Review: Vegetables and Fruit in the Prevention of Chronic Diseases, *European Journal of Nutrition*, 51, no. 5 (2012):637–63.

63 Pieter Van't Veer, et al, "Fruits and Vegetables in the Prevention of Cancer and Cardiovascular Disease," *Public Health Nutrition* 3.1 (2000): 103–107.

64 Lydia A. Bazzano, Mary K. Serdula, and Simin Liu, "Dietary Intake of Fruits and Vegetables and Risk of Cardiovascular Disease," *Current Atherosclerosis Reports* 5.6 (2003): 492–499.

65 A. R. Ness, J. W. Fowles, "Fruit and Vegetables and Cardiovascular Disease: A Review." *International Journal of Epidemiology* 26 (1997): 1–13.

66 Earl S. Ford and Ali H. Mokdad, "Fruit and Vegetable Consumption and Diabetes Mellitus Incidence among US Adults." *Preventive Medicine* 32.1 (2001): 33–39. Also see Feskens EJ, Virtanen SM, Rasanen L, Tuomilehto J, Stengard J, Pekkanen J, Nissinen A, Kromhout D "Dietary Factors Determining Diabetes and Impaired Glucose Tolerance: a 20-year Follow-up of the Finnish and Dutch Cohorts of the Seven Countries Study. *Diabetes Care* 18:1104–1112, 1995.

67 K. He, F. B. Hu, G. A. Colditz, J. E. Manson, W. C. Willett, and S. Liu, "Changes in Intake of Fruits and Vegetables in Relation to Risk of Obesity and Weight Gain among Middle-Aged Women," *International Journal of Obesity* 28, no. 12 (2004): 1569–1574.

68 T. Colin Campbell and Thomas M. Campbell, *The China Study: The Most Comprehensive Study of Nutrition Ever Conducted and the Startling Implications for Diet, Weight Loss, and Long-Term Health* (Wakefield Press, 2007).

69 Jeanine M. Genkinger and Anita Koushik, "Meat Consumption and Cancer Risk," *PLOS Medicine* 4, no. 12 (2007): e345.

70 Amanda J. Cross, Michael F. Leitzmann, Mitchell H. Gail, Albert R. Hollenbeck, Arthur Schatzkin, and Rashmi Sinha, "A Prospective Study of Red and Processed Meat Intake in Relation to Cancer Risk," *PLOS Medicine* 4, no. 12 (2007): e325.

71 T. Colin Campbell and Thomas M. Campbell, *The China Study*, 59.

72 Artemis P. Simopoulos, "The Importance of the Ratio of Omega-6/Omega-3 Essential Fatty Acids," *Biomedicine & Pharmacotherapy* 56, no. 8 (2002): 365–379.

73   Artemis P. Simopoulos, "The Importance of the Omega-6/Omega-3
      Fatty Acid Ratio in Cardiovascular Disease and Other Chronic Diseases,"
      Experimental Biology and Medicine 233, no. 6 (2008): 674–688.

74   Qi Sun, Jing Ma, Hannia Campos, Susan E. Hankinson, JoAnn E. Manson,
      Meir J. Stampfer, Kathryn M. Rexrode, Walter C. Willett, and Frank B.
      Hu, "A Prospective Study of Trans Fatty Acids in Erythrocytes and Risk of
      Coronary Heart Disease," *Circulation* 115, no. 14 (2007): 1858–1865.

75   C. M. Oomen, M. C. Ocke, E. J. Feskens, M. A. van Erp-Baart, F. J. Kok,
      D. Kromhout. "Association between Trans-Fatty Acid Intake and 10-Year
      Risk of Coronary Heart Disease in the Zutphen Elderly Study: A Prospective
      Population-Based Study," *Lancet* 357 (2001): 746–751.

76   R. P. M. Mensink, M. B. Katan, "Effect of Dietary Trans-Fatty Acids on
      High-Density and Low-Density Lipoprotein Cholesterol Levels in Healthy
      Subjects," *New England Journal of Medicine* 323 (1990): 439–45.

77   Steen Stender, Jørn Dyerberg, and Arne Astrup, "High Levels of Industrially
      Produced Trans Fat in Popular Fast Foods," *New England Journal of Medicine*
      354, no. 15 (2006): 1650–1652.

78   Strategies to Reduce Sodium Intake in the United States, Institute of
      Medicine, April 2010 http://www.iom.edu/~/media/Files/Report%20
      Files/2010/Strategies-to-Reduce-Sodium-Intake-in-the-United-States/
      Strategies%20to%20Reduce%20Sodium%20Intake%202010%20%20
      Report%20Brief.ashx

79   Kathryn E. Wellen and Gökhan S. Hotamisligil, "Inflammation, Stress, and
      Diabetes," *Journal of Clinical Investigation* 115, no. 5 (2005): 1111–1119.

80   Göran K. Hansson, "Inflammation, Atherosclerosis, and Coronary Artery
      Disease," *New England Journal of Medicine* 352, no. 16 (2005): 1685–1695.

81   Marta Scatena, Lucy Liaw, and Cecilia M. Giachelli, "Osteopontin and
      Multifunctional Molecule Regulating Chronic Inflammation and Vascular
      Disease," *Arteriosclerosis, Thrombosis, and Vascular Biology* 27, no. 11 (2007):
      2302–2309.

82   See http://www.melissadianesmith.com/Articles/WheatGlutenSensitivity.
      html

83   Melissa Smith, *Going Against the Grain: How Reducing and Avoiding Grains
      Can Revitalize Your Health* (Contemporary Books, 2002).

84   Melissa Smith, *Going Against the Grain: How Reducing and Avoiding Grains
      Can Revitalize Your Health* (Contemporary Books, 2002).

85   See http://www.huffingtonpost.com/dr-mark-hyman/wheat-gluten_b_1274872.html.

86   Kelly McGonical, *The Neuroscience of Change: A Compassion-Based Program for Personal Transformation*, audio course (Sounds True, 2012).

87   Kelly McGonigal, *The Willpower Instinct: How Self-Control Works, Why It Matters, and What You Can Do to Get More of It* (Avery, 2012).

88   Lars Schwabe, Oliver Höffken, Martin Tegenthoff, and Oliver T. Wolf, "Preventing the Stress-Induced Shift from Goal-Directed to Habit Action with a β-Adrenergic Antagonist," *The Journal of Neuroscience* 31, no. 47 (2011): 17317–17325.

89   A. F. Arnsten, "Stress Signalling Pathways That Impair Prefrontal Cortex Structure and Function," Nature Reviews Neuroscience 10, no. 6 (2009): 410–422.

90   S. Gottfried, *The Hormone Cure,* (Scribner, 2013).

91   S. Gottfried, *The Hormone Cure.*

92   M. Hyman, *The UltraMind Solution* (Scribner, 2009).

93   See http://www.apa.org/news/press/releases/stress/2012/full-report.pdf.

94   Olivia Longe, Frances A. Maratos, Paul Gilbert, Gaynor Evans, Faye Volker, Helen Rockliff, and Gina Rippon, "Having a Word with Yourself: Neural Correlates of Self-Criticism and Self-Reassurance," *Neuroimage* 49, no. 2 (2010): 1849–1856.

95   A. K. I. N. Ahmet and Yapısal Eşitlik Modeliyle Bir İnceleme, "Self-Compassion and Achievement Goals: A Structural Equation Modeling Approach." Also see Theodore A. Powers, Richard Koestner, David C. Zuroff, Marina Milyavskaya, and Amy A. Gorin, "The Effects of Self-Criticism and Self-Oriented Perfectionism on Goal Pursuit," *Personality and Social Psychology Bulletin* 37, no. 7 (2011): 964–975.

96   Bayram Çetin, Hasan Basri Gündüz, and Ahmet Akın. "An Investigation of the Relationships between Self-Compassion, Motivation, and Burnout with Structural Equation Modeling [English]," *Abant İzzet Baysal Üniversitesi Eğitim Fakültesi Dergisi* (2008).

97   Olivia Longe, Frances A. Maratos, Paul Gilbert, Gaynor Evans, Faye Volker, Helen Rockliff, and Gina Rippon, "Having a Word with Yourself: Neural Correlates of Self-Criticism and Self-Reassurance," *Neuroimage* 49, no. 2 (2010): 1849–1856.

98   Kristin D. Neff, Stephanie S. Rude, and Kristin L. Kirkpatrick, "An Examination of Self-Compassion in Relation to Positive Psychological Functioning and Personality Traits," *Journal of Research in Personality* 41, no. 4 (2007): 908–916.

99   Olivia Longe, Frances A. Maratos, Paul Gilbert, Gaynor Evans, Faye Volker, Helen Rockliff, and Gina Rippon, "Having a Word with Yourself: Neural Correlates of Self-Criticism and Self-Reassurance," *Neuroimage* 49, no. 2 (2010): 1849–1856.

100 Kristin Neff, "Self-Compassion," in *Handbook of Individual Differences in Social Behavior*, ed. M. R. Leary and R. H. Hoyle (Guilford Press, 2009), 561–73.

101 See http://www.self-compassion.org/what-is-self-compassion/the-three-elements-of-self-compassion.html.

102 Claire E. Adams and Mark R. Leary, "Promoting Self-Compassionate Attitudes toward Eating among Restrictive and Guilty Eaters," *Journal of Social and Clinical Psychology* 26, no. 10 (2007): 1120–1144.

103 Kelly McGonigal, *The Willpower Instinct*, 148.

104 Claire E. Adams and Mark R. Leary, "Promoting Self-Compassionate Attitudes toward Eating among Restrictive and Guilty Eaters," *Journal of Social and Clinical Psychology* 26, no. 10 (2007): 1120–1144.

105 Jean Fain, *The Self-Compassion Diet: A Step-by-Step Program to Lose Weight with Loving-Kindness* (Sounds True, 2011). Also see http://www.self-compassion.org.

106 Claire E. Adams and Mark R. Leary, "Promoting Self-Compassionate Attitudes toward Eating among Restrictive and Guilty Eaters," *Journal of Social and Clinical Psychology* 26, no. 10 (2007): 1120–1144.

107 Stephen Covey, *The 7 Habits of Highly Effective People* (Simon & Schuster, 1989), 102.

108 Gabriele Oettingen and Peter M. Gollwitzer, *Strategies of Setting and Implementing Goals: Mental Contrasting and Implementation Intentions,* Bibliothek der Universität Konstanz, 2010.

109 Peter M. Gollwitzer, "Implementation Intentions: Strong Effects of Simple Plans," *American Psychologist* 54, no. 7 (1999): 493.

110 Gertraud Stadler, Gabriele Oettingen, and Peter M. Gollwitzer, "Physical Activity in Women: Effects of a Self-Regulation Intervention," *American Journal of Preventive Medicine* 36, no. 1 (2009): 29–34.

111   "URI Researcher Provides Further Evidence That Slow Eating Reduces Food Intake," University of Rhode Island, Media Release, October 27, 2011, http://www.uri.edu/news/releases/?id=6019.

112   Deborah Kesten, *The Healing Secrets of Food: A Practical Guide for Nourishing Body, Mind, and Soul* (New World Library, 2001)

113   Brian Wansink, Collin Payne, Pierre Chandon, "Internal and External Cues of Meal Cessation: The French Paradox Redux?" *North American Association for the Study of Obesity* 12, no. 12 (2007): 2920–2924.

114   The Brain: How the Brain Rewires Itself, Sharon Begley, Time Magazine, Friday, January 19th, 2007. http://palousemindfulness.com/docs/brain-rewires.pdf

115   Lisa Morrone, *Overcoming Overeating: It's Not What You Eat, It's What's Eating You!* (Harvest House, 2009).

116   To further explore the concepts of vital nerve energy, please refer to Dr. T. C. Fry's e-book *Raw Energy Mini-Course: Seven Special Lessons in How to Naturally Supercharge Yourself with Energy and Transform Your Life.* Republished with permission by David Klein, 2010.

117   Douglas Graham, *The 80/10/10 Diet*, 80.

118   David C. Jimerson, Michael D. Lesem, Walter H. Kaye, Arlene P. Hegg, and Timothy D. Brewerton, "Eating Disorders and Depression: Is There a Serotonin Connection?" *Biological Psychiatry* 28, no. 5 (1990): 443–454.

119   Anne Katherine, *Anatomy of a Food Addiction*.

120   E. Baron Short, Samet Kose, Qiwen Mu, Jeffery Borckardt, Andrew Newberg, Mark S. George, and F. Andrew Kozel, "Regional Brain Activation during Meditation Shows Time and Practice Effects: An Exploratory FMRI Study," *Evidence-Based Complementary and Alternative Medicine* 7, no. 1 (2010): 121–127. Also see the following: Yi-Yuan Tang, Yinghua Ma, Junhong Wang, Yaxin Fan, Shigang Feng, Qilin Lu, and Qingbao Yu, et al, "Short-Term Meditation Training Improves Attention and Self-Regulation," *Proceedings of the National Academy of Sciences* 104, no. 43 (2007): 17152–17156. Fadel Zeidan, Susan K. Johnson, Bruce J. Diamond, Zhanna David, and Paula Goolkasian. "Mindfulness Meditation Improves Cognition: Evidence of Brief Mental Training," *Consciousness and Cognition* 19, no. 2 (2010): 597–605. Kirk Warren Brown and Richard M. Ryan, "The Benefits of Being Present: Mindfulness and Its Role in Psychological Well-Being," *Journal of Personality and Social Psychology* 84, no. 4 (2003): 822.

121 E. Luder, A. W. Toga, N. Lepore, and C. Gaser, "The Underlying Anatomical Correlates of Long-Term Meditation: Larger Hippocampal and Frontal Volumes of Grey Matter," *Neuroimage* 45, no. 3 (2009): 672–678.

122 Jean L. Kristeller and Ruth Q. Wolever, "Mindfulness-Based Eating Awareness Training for Treating Binge Eating Disorder: The Conceptual Foundation," *Eating Disorders* 19, no. 1 (2010): 49–61.

123 Troels W. Kjaer, Camilla Bertelsen, Paola Piccini, David Brooks, Jørgen Alving, and Hans C. Lou, "Increased Dopamine Tone during Meditation-Induced Change of Consciousness," *Cognitive Brain Research* 13, no. 2 (2002): 255–259.

124 Mahmoud Hosseini, Hojjat Allah Alaei, Asieh Naderi, Mohammad Reza Sharifi, and Reza Zahed, "Treadmill Exercise Reduces Self-Administration of Morphine in Male Rats," *Pathophysiology* 16, no. 1 (2009): 3–7.

125 Arthur F. Kramer and Kirk I. Erickson, "Capitalizing on Cortical Plasticity: Influence of Physical Activity on Cognition and Brain Function," *Trends in Cognitive Sciences* 11, no. 8 (2007): 342–348. Also see Henriette van Praag, "Exercise and the Brain: Something to Chew On," *Trends in Neurosciences* 32, no. 5 (2009): 283–290.

126 Valorie N. Salimpoor, Mitchel Benovoy, Kevin Larcher, Alain Dagher, and Robert J. Zatorre, "Anatomically Distinct Dopamine Release during Anticipation and Experience of Peak Emotion to Music," *Nature Neuroscience* 14, no. 2 (2011): 257–262.

127 Brian Wansink and Collin Payne, "Why Exercise Makes Us Fat: Compensation between Physical Activity and Food Consumption," *Building Connections* 39 (2011): 506.

128 Harvey R. Colten and Bruce M. Altevogt, eds., *Sleep Disorders and Sleep Deprivation: An Unmet Public Health Problem* (National Academies Press, 2006).

129 Matthew P. Walker and Els van Der Helm, "Overnight Therapy? The Role of Sleep in Emotional Brain Processing," *Psychological Bulletin* 135, no. 5 (2009): 731–748.

130 Yasmin Anwar, "Sleep Loss Linked to Psychiatric Disorders," *UC Berkeley News* press release, October 2007, http://berkeley.edu/news/media/releases/2007/10/22_sleeploss.shtml.

131 Kristen L. Knutson, Karine Spiegel, Plamen Penev, and Eve Van Cauter. "The Metabolic Consequences of Sleep Deprivation," *Sleep Medicine Reviews* 11, no. 3 (2007): 163–178.

132 Harvey R. Colten and Bruce M. Altevogt, eds., *Sleep Disorders and Sleep Deprivation: An Unmet Public Health Problem.*

133 "Lack of Sleep May Increase Calorie Consumption," American Heart Association, March 14, 2012, http://newsroom.heart.org/news/lack-of-sleep-may-increase-calorie-230068.

134 Shahrad Taheri, Ling Lin, Diane Austin, Terry Young, and Emmanuel Mignot, "Short Sleep Duration Is Associated with Reduced Leptin, Elevated Ghrelin, and Increased Body Mass Index," *PLOS Medicine* 1, no. 3 (2004): e62.

135 Karine Spiegel, Kristen Knutson, Rachel Leproult, Esra Tasali, and Eve Van Cauter, "Sleep Loss: A Novel Risk Factor for Insulin Resistance and Type 2 Diabetes," *Journal of Applied Physiology* 99, no. 5 (2005): 2008–2019.

136 See http://www.drnorthrup.com/womenshealth/healthcenter/topic_details.php?topic_id=114.

137 See Institute of Heart Math website: http://www.heartmath.org

138 Rollin McCraty, "Science of the Heart: Exploring the Role of the Heart in Human Performance: An Overview of Research Conducted by the Institute of HeartMath," 2001, www.heartmath.org.

139 Nathaniel Altman, *The Little Giant Encyclopedia of Meditations & Blessings* (Sterling Publishing, 2000).